Pediatric Oral and Maxillofacial Pathology

Editors

ANTONIA KOLOKYTHAS
MICHAEL MILORO

ORAL AND MAXILLOFACIAL SURGERY CLINICS OF NORTH AMERICA

www.oralmaxsurgery.theclinics.com

Consulting Editor
RICHARD H. HAUG

February 2016 • Volume 28 • Number 1

ELSEVIER

1600 John F. Kennedy Boulevard ● Suite 1800 ● Philadelphia, Pennsylvania, 19103-2899

http://www.oralmaxsurgery.theclinics.com

ORAL AND MAXILLOFACIAL SURGERY CLINICS OF NORTH AMERICA Volume 28, Number 1
February 2016 ISSN 1042-3699, ISBN-13: 978-0-323-41704-4

Editor: John Vassallo; j.vassallo@elsevier.com
Developmental Editor: Colleen Viola

Oral and Maxillofacial Surgery Clinics of North America (ISSN 1042-3699) is published quarterly by Elsevier Inc., 360 Park Avenue South, New York, NY 10010-1710. Months of issue are February, May, August, and November. Business and Editorial Offices: 1600 John F. Kennedy Blvd., Suite 1800, Philadelphia, PA 19103-2899. Periodicals postage paid at New York, NY and additional mailing offices. Subscription prices are $385.00 per year for US individuals, $628.00 per year for US institutions, $100.00 per year for US students and residents, $455.00 per year for Canadian individuals, $753.00 per year for Canadian institutions, $520.00 per year for international individuals, $753.00 per year for international institutions and $235.00 per year for Canadian and foreign students/residents. To receive student/resident rate, orders must be accompanied by name of affiliated institution, date of term, and the *signature* of program/residency coordinator on institution letterhead. Orders will be billed at individual rate until proof of status is received. Foreign air speed delivery is included in all *Clinics* subscription prices. All prices are subject to change without notice. **POSTMASTER:** Send address changes to *Oral and Maxillofacial Surgery Clinics of North America,* Elsevier Periodicals **Customer Service, 11830 Westline Industrial Drive, St. Louis, MO 63146. Tel: 1-800-654-2452 (U.S. and Canada); 314-447-8871 (outside U.S. and Canada). Fax: 314-447-8029. E-mail: journals customerservice-usa@elsevier.com (for print support); journalsonlinesupport-usa@elsevier.com (for online support).**

Reprints. For copies of 100 or more, of articles in this publication, please contact the Commercial Reprints Department, Elsevier Inc., 360 Park Avenue South, New York, NY 10010-1710. Tel.: 212-633-3874; Fax: 212-633-3820; Email: reprints@elsevier.com.

Oral and Maxillofacial Surgery Clinics of North America is covered in *MEDLINE/PubMed (Index Medicus)*, *Science Citation Index Expanded (SciSearch®)*, *Journal Citation Reports/Science Edition*, and *Current Contents®/Clinical Medicine*.

Contributors

CONSULTING EDITOR

RICHARD H. HAUG, DDS
Professor and Chief, Oral Maxillofacial Surgery, Carolinas Medical Center, Charlotte, North Carolina

EDITORS

ANTONIA KOLOKYTHAS, DDS, MSc
Department Head and Program Director, Oral and Maxillofacial Surgery, University of Rochester, Strong Memorial Hospital-EIOH, Rochester, New York

MICHAEL MILORO, DMD, MD, FACS
Professor and Head, Department of Oral and Maxillofacial Surgery, University of Illinois at Chicago, Chicago, Illinois

AUTHORS

JOSHUA M. ABRAHAMS, DMD
Former Chief Resident, Department of Oral and Maxillofacial Surgery, Broward Health Medical Center, Nova Southeastern University College of Dental Medicine, Ft. Lauderdale, Florida; Private Practice, Long Island Oral and Maxillofacial Surgery, Mineola, New York

KEVIN ARCE, DMD, MD, MCR
Assistant Professor of Surgery and Residency Program Director, Division of Oral and Maxillofacial Surgery, Department of Surgery, Mayo College of Medicine, Mayo Clinic, Rochester, Minnesota

NAWAF ASLAM-PERVEZ, DDS, MD
Senior Resident, Department of Oral Maxillofacial Surgery, University of Maryland School of Dentistry, Baltimore, Maryland

CARL BOUCHARD, DMD, MSc, FRCD(C)
Assistant Professor of Oral and Maxillofacial Surgery, Hôpital de l'Enfant-Jésus, Centre Hospitalier Universitaire de Québec, Laval University, Québec, Québec, Canada

ERIC R. CARLSON, DMD, MD, FACS
Professor and Kelly L. Krahwinkel Chairman, Department of Oral and Maxillofacial Surgery; Director, Oral and Maxillofacial Surgery Residency Program; Director, Oral/Head and Neck Oncologic Surgery Fellowship Program, University of Tennessee Medical Center, University of Tennessee Cancer Institute, Knoxville, Tennessee

DANIEL K. CHOI, MD, MS
Instructor of Pediatrics, Division of Pediatric Hematology/Oncology, Department of Pediatrics, University of Illinois at Chicago College of Medicine, Chicago, Illinois

PHILIP P. CONNELL, MD
Associate Professor, Department of Radiation and Cellular Oncology, University of Chicago Medical Center, Chicago, Illinois

JASJIT DILLON, MBBS, DDS, FDSRCS, FACS
Clinical Associate Professor, Department of Oral and Maxillofacial Surgery; Residency Program Director, Acting Chief of Service, Harborview Medical Center, School of Dentistry, University of Washington, Seattle, Washington

DONITA DYALRAM, DDS, MD, FACS
Assistant Professor and Associate Program Director, Department of Oral Maxillofacial Surgery, University of Maryland School of Dentistry, Baltimore, Maryland

ISSAM EID, MD
Assistant Professor, Department of Otolaryngology, University of Mississippi Medical Center, Jackson, Mississippi

KYLE S. ETTINGER, DDS, MD
Resident, Division of Oral and Maxillofacial Surgery, Department of Surgery, Mayo College of Medicine, Mayo Clinic, Rochester, Minnesota

ALEXANDRA GLICKMAN, DDS
Resident, Oral and Maxillofacial Surgery, New York University-Bellevue Hospital Center, New York, New York

RICHARD SCOTT JONES, DDS
Resident, Department of Oral and Maxillofacial Surgery, University of Washington, Seattle, Washington

VASILIKI KARLIS, DMD, MD, FACS
Associate Professor and Director of Advanced Education Program, Oral and Maxillofacial Surgery, New York University-Bellevue Hospital Center, New York, New York

ANTONIA KOLOKYTHAS, DDS, MSc
Department Head and Program Director, Oral and Maxillofacial Surgery, University of Rochester, Strong Memorial Hospital-EIOH, Rochester, New York

JOSHUA E. LUBEK, DDS, MD, FACS
Assistant Professor and Fellowship Director, Department of Oral Maxillofacial Surgery, University of Maryland School of Dentistry, Baltimore, Maryland

SHAWN A. McCLURE, DMD, MD, FACS
Residency Program Director, Director of Research, Associate Professor, Department of Oral and Maxillofacial Surgery, Broward Health Medical Center, Nova Southeastern University College of Dental Medicine, Ft. Lauderdale, Florida

ROBERT A. ORD, DDS, MD, FRCS, FACS, MS, MBA
Professor and Chairman, Department of Oral and Maxillofacial Surgery, Baltimore College of Dental Surgery, University of Maryland and the Greenebaum Cancer Institute, Baltimore, Maryland

ZACHARY S. PEACOCK, DMD, MD
Department of Oral and Maxillofacial Surgery, Massachusetts General Hospital, Boston, Massachusetts

MOHAMMED QAISI, DMD, MD
Assistant Professor, Department of Oral and Maxillofacial Surgery; Adjunct Assistant Professor, Department of Otolaryngology, University of Mississippi Medical Center, Jackson, Mississippi

MARY LOU SCHMIDT, MD
Professor of Pediatrics, Division of Pediatric Hematology/Oncology, Department of Pediatrics, University of Illinois at Chicago College of Medicine, Chicago, Illinois

MICHAEL T. SPIOTTO, MD, PhD
Assistant Professor, Department of Radiation and Cellular Oncology, University of Chicago Medical Center; Lecturer, Department of Radiation Oncology, University of Illinois at Chicago Medical Center, Chicago, Illinois

CHRISTOPHER S. STREFF, DDS, MD
Resident, Division of Oral and Maxillofacial Surgery, Department of Surgery, Mayo College of Medicine, Mayo Clinic, Rochester, Minnesota

MARIA J. TROULIS, DDS, MSc
Chief of Service Oral and Maxillofacial Surgery, Massachusetts General Hospital, Walter C. Guralnick Professor and Chair of Oral and Maxillofacial Surgery, Harvard School of Dental Medicine, Boston, Massachusetts

Contents

Despite the many types of oral pathologic lesions found in infants and children, the most commonly encountered are benign soft tissue lesions. The clinical features, diagnostic criteria, and treatment algorithms of pathologies in the age group from birth to 18 years of age are summarized based on their prevalence in each given age distribution. Treatment modalities include both medical and surgical management.

Head and neck malignancies are rare in pediatric patients and represent 12% of all pediatric malignancies. The incidence for these head and neck tumors is 1.49 cases per 1,000,000 person-years. Among the most common pediatric head and neck malignancies are lymphomas (27%), neural tumors including primitive neurectodermal tumors (23%), thyroid malignancies (21%), soft tissue sarcomas including rhabdomyosarcoma (12%), nasopharyngeal carcinoma, skeletal and odontogenic malignancies including osteosarcoma, Ewing sarcoma, and ameloblastic carcinoma. This article presents an overview of pediatric head and neck malignancies with emphasis on diagnosis and management.

Odontogenic cysts represent a common form of pathology of the jaws, and the natural history, clinicopathologic findings, and appropriate management strategies are important to the oral and maxillofacial surgeon. Odontogenic cysts in the pediatric populations are important pathologic entities given their potential impact on the growth and development of the maxillofacial complex. Inappropriate management strategies can severely affect the form and function of the growing child. Categorizing pediatric odontogenic cysts into inflammatory or developmental causes provides a convenient way of conceptualizing these various entities and helps facilitate the appropriate diagnosis and the subsequent management.

Nonodontogenic cysts within the jaws are not a common presentation in the pediatric population. Cysts within the pediatric population tend to be developmental and odontogenic in nature. Although nonodontogenic cysts of the jaws are relatively uncommon, it is imperative that the clinician understands their clinical behavior and management, because failure to do so can result in increased patient morbidity. The nonodontogenic cysts of the jaws that are most often encountered are the central giant cell granuloma, traumatic bone cavity, aneurysmal bone cyst, nasopalatine duct cyst, and nasolabial cyst. This article reviews common clinical findings, radiographic features, histopathologic features, and current treatments of nonodontogenic cysts.

by an inconsistency in the nomenclature for these lesions found in the literature. This article covers the clinical presentation, etiology, and pathophysiology and treatment approaches of the vascular anomalies in the pediatric population.

Oral and maxillofacial surgeons are often involved in the diagnosis and treatment of vascular neoplasms of the head and neck. An incorrect diagnosis may lead to improper or unnecessary treatment. This article reviews the diagnosis and management of vascular tumors.

Most pediatric head and neck cancers are treated with radiotherapy, but the morbidity associated with radiotherapy has become a prominent issue. This article discusses the common long-term complications associated with head and neck radiotherapy for childhood cancers. It reviews approaches to minimize toxicity and details the toxicities that head and neck radiation inflicts on relevant functional measures. In addition, it discusses the risk of radiation-induced secondary cancers in childhood cancer survivors, as well as strategies to reduce them. Thus, this article addresses approaches to minimize long-term radiation toxicities in order to improve the quality of life for childhood cancer survivors.

Cancers of the head and neck in children represent a heterogeneous group of malignancies requiring a variety of treatment modalities. In many instances of childhood head and neck cancers, chemotherapy will be required for treatment, often in conjunction with surgery and/or radiation therapy. Chemotherapy in children with head and neck cancers poses unique challenges in terms of immediate as well as long-term toxicities. This article focuses on the common chemotherapeutic agents, with a particular focus on early and late effects, used in the treatment of children with head and neck cancers.

ORAL AND MAXILLOFACIAL SURGERY CLINICS OF NORTH AMERICA

FORTHCOMING ISSUES

May 2016
Management of the Cleft Patient
Kevin S. Smith, *Editor*

August 2016
Oral and Maxillofacial Pain
Steven J. Scrivani, *Editor*

November 2016
Coagulopathy
Jeffrey D. Bennett and Elie M. Ferneini,
Editors

RECENT ISSUES

November 2015
**Management of Medication-related
Osteonecrosis of the Jaw**
Salvatore L. Ruggiero, *Editor*

August 2015
Dentoalveolar Surgery
Michael A. Kleiman, *Editor*

May 2015
Dental Implants: An Evolving Discipline
Alex M. Greenberg, *Editor*

RELATED INTEREST

Dental Clinics of North America
October 2014 (Vol. 58, No. 4)
Geriatric Dentistry
Lisa A. Thompson and Leonard J. Brennan, *Editors*
Available at: www.dental.theclinics.com

THE CLINICS ARE NOW AVAILABLE ONLINE!
Access your subscription at:
www.theclinics.com

Preface
Current Therapy in Pediatric Oral and Maxillofacial Pathology

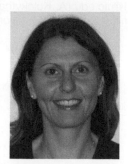
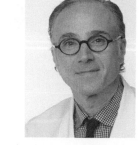

Antonia Kolokythas, DDS, MSc   Michael Miloro, DMD, MD, FACS
Editors

The soul is healed by being with children.
—Fyodor Dostoyevsky

All parents set out with expectations, hopes and dreams for their child. When a child is diagnosed with a health problem, these aspirations are altered. While one parent is hoping to see their child graduate from a university, another is praying that they can live pain free.
—Sharon Dempsey, 2008

Perhaps no area of Oral and Maxillofacial Surgery invokes such impassioned and attentive concern by the clinician as does the diagnosis and management of the pediatric patient with a health problem, because we believe inherently that children represent a pure and clean subset of the human race that should be exposed only to the positive aspects of life and should not be affected by the negative influences that typically plague adults, principally during the advanced stages of life after having lived a long, significant, fruitful, and worthwhile life. Other than for elective prophylactic care, it is generally accepted that a child does not belong in a clinic or a hospital setting, since these impersonal institutional locations represent places where the sick and infirm are evaluated and treated

with medications, radiation therapy, and surgery. Children represent our future, and it is a tragedy to be a witness to the possibility that the future of our species may be in jeopardy due to a health-related illness. It is therefore significant when a child with a benign, or worse, malignant lesion presents for care that the entire health care team takes special notice and provides their utmost and focused attention. It is the primary intention of the management team to eradicate the problem in this group of patients as soon as possible to return them to their care-free lives of happiness and joy.

This issue is devoted to those children who have the unfortunate occurrence of a lesion of the head and neck region that requires multidisciplinary management by a team of experts with advanced experience and training, and the most recent evidence-based advances in diagnosis and management at their disposal to most appropriately and efficiently diagnose, provide treatment, and eradicate the problem. The authors selected for this issue are recognized experts in these areas of head and neck pathology, and they provide the most current available options in the assessment and treatment of the child with oral and maxillofacial pathology. These excellent articles stress the importance of a team approach to these

Oral Maxillofacial Surg Clin N Am 28 (2016) ix–x
http://dx.doi.org/10.1016/j.coms.2015.10.001
1042-3699/16/$ – see front matter © 2016 Published by Elsevier Inc.

lesions in order to most effectively manage these patients and to preserve our future.

Antonia Kolokythas, DDS, MSc
Department of Oral and Maxillofacial Surgery
University of Rochester
Strong Memorial Hospital-EIOH
601 Elmwood Ave, AC-4
Rochester, NY 14642, USA

Michael Miloro, DMD, MD, FACS
Department of Oral and Maxillofacial Surgery
University of Illinois at Chicago
801 South Paulina Street
Room 110
Chicago, IL 60612, USA

E-mail addresses:
ga1@uic.edu (A. Kolokythas)
mmiloro@uic.edu (M. Miloro)

Pediatric Benign Soft Tissue Oral and Maxillofacial Pathology

Alexandra Glickman, DDS[1], Vasiliki Karlis, DMD, MD*

KEYWORDS

- Pediatric • Oral surgery • Oral pathology • Neoplasms • Oral biopsy • Oral diagnosis

KEY POINTS

- Pediatric oral and maxillofacial pathologies are typically categorized by presenting age group.
- Most pediatric pathologies are benign or secondary to soft tissue trauma.
- Because of their benign nature, management is straightforward, usually palliation or simple surgical excision.

Several oral lesions, systemic manifestations, and soft tissue pathologies occur in the pediatric population. Many of these are unique in that they correlate with specific definable age groups. These presentations are significant in that the period from birth to adolescence is the most dynamic period of growth and development, and small changes have the capacity for long-lasting impact. It is also a sensitive time for both child and parent. Fortunately, most pediatric pathology is benign and does not require extensive surgical intervention. In a study performed by Jones and Franklin,[1] over the course of a 30-year period, only 1% of pathologic specimens submitted for children 16 years and younger were found to be malignant. This article discusses the most common types of benign pediatric soft tissue pathologies based on age range, including their clinical appearance, diagnostic features, and treatment algorithms (**Box 1**).

NEONATES/INFANTS
Newborn Palatal Cyst

It is common to find developmental palatal cysts in the newborn. Usually they present as asymptomatic 1 to 3 mm, white-yellowish papules that appear along the palatal midline. They frequently occur in clusters, however, they can also occur as single lesions. Two common examples are Epstein pearls and Bohn nodules. Epstein pearls are found in approximately 75% to 80% of newborns. They occur along the median palatal raphe and arise from epithelium that is trapped along the line of fusion of the palatal shelves during embryogenesis. Bohn nodules, also common, occur on the palate of newborns, likely from developing minor salivary glands. They are usually found on the buccal and lingual aspects of the ridge, removed from the midline. Histologically, both are keratin-filled cysts. As a result, they require no treatment and usually resolve on their own within the first 3 months of life.[2–4]

Hemangioma

Hemangiomas are the most common congenital vascular tumors of infancy, with highest incidence in white women.[5] They are usually noticed within the first 2 months after birth as bright red raised lesions that are firm and rubbery to palpation, comparable with the texture and appearance of a

Financial Disclosure: V. Karlis has Royalty Agreement with Stryker Craniofacial. A. Glickman has nothing to disclose.

Oral and Maxillofacial Surgery, New York University-Bellevue Hospital Center, New York, NY, USA
[1] 550 1st Avenue, New York, NY 10016, USA
* Corresponding author. Department of Oral and Maxillofacial Surgery, NYU College of Dentistry, 345 East 24th Street, Room 201, New York, NY 10010.
E-mail address: vk1@nyu.edu

Oral Maxillofacial Surg Clin N Am 28 (2016) 1–10
http://dx.doi.org/10.1016/j.coms.2015.07.005
1042-3699/16/$ – see front matter

Box 1
Common pediatric benign soft tissue lesions

Neonates/Infants

Newborn palatal cysts

  Epstein pearls

  Bohn nodules

Hemangiomas

Lymphangiomas

Congenital epulis

Melanotic neuroectodermal tumor of infancy

Age 2 y and Older

Fibroma

Pyogenic granuloma

Peripheral giant cell granuloma

Peripheral ossifying fibroma

Parulis

Eruption Cyst/Eruption Hematoma

Mucocele

Gingival hyperplasia

  Inflammatory

  Medication-induced

  Spongiotic

  Idiopathic

  Leukemic infiltrates

Recurrent aphthous ulcers

Herpes simplex virus

  Primary

  Recurrent

Macroglossia

Ankyloglossia

Soft tissue anesthesia trauma

---

strawberry. Sixty percent of these occur in the head and neck, 80% of which are solitary lesions. Their distribution generally correlates with regions of embryologic fusion.[6] During the subsequent 6- to 10-month period, they reach their peak growth period and begin to involute. About half of all hemangiomas completely resolve by age 5 years and 90% resolve by age 9 years. As a result, treatment usually consists of observation only. When the lesion is in a region that could cause local or life-threatening complications, medicaments are the treatment of choice. Systemic steroids have been shown to reduce the size of larger hemangiomas, with a 70% to 90% response rate.

Intralesional steroids, topical steroids, and sclerosing agents have been shown to be efficacious for smaller localized lesions. Intravenously administered vincristine can be used for complicated tumors that are unresponsive to systemic steroids.[2] Most recently, topical nanopropranolol has been introduced as a treatment modality for hemangiomas as well.[6]

Lymphangioma

Lymphangiomas, also known as cystic hygromas and lymphatic malformations, are benign tumors of the lymphatic vessels. They are believed to be malformations that arise from portions of lymphatic tissue that do not communicate normally with the rest of the lymphatic system.[2] Seventy-five percent occur in the head and neck region, which harbors the body's richest lymphatic bed.[7] Half of all lesions are noted at birth and about 90% develop by 2 years of age. Large lymphangiomas can often lead to airway compromise, and therefore treatment usually consists of sclerotherapy and surgical removal. In cases where it is not possible to remove the entire tumor because of proximity to vital structures, tracheostomy is used to secure the airway, and ultimately, serial debulking procedures are performed to reduce the size of the lymphangioma (**Fig. 1**).[8]

Congenital Epulis (Congenital Epulis of the Newborn; Congenital Granular Cell Lesion)

This is a more uncommon pathologic lesion that occurs almost exclusively on the alveolar ridges of newborns, most commonly seen in girls. Clinically it appears as a distinct polypoid mass of tissue that is similar in color and consistency to normal mucosa. Generally, they are less than 2 cm in size, but can interfere with normal respiration or feeding, even though 90% of the time they occur in the anterior maxilla at the lateral incisor-cuspid region.[2,3]

Treatment is surgical excision of the epulis, and even with incomplete removal, these masses have not been shown to recur.[2] If necessary due to excessive size, they can be excised hours to days after birth under general or local anesthesia, or in some cases during the actual delivery, if the lesion was identified in utero.[9–11]

Melanotic Neuroectodermal Tumor of Infancy

These tumors are extremely rare, but they are seen in the infant population; 82% of the time these tumors occur in infants less than 6 months old, with a slight predilection for boys. They most frequently occur in the maxillofacial region, including the maxilla (68%–80%), skull (10.8%),

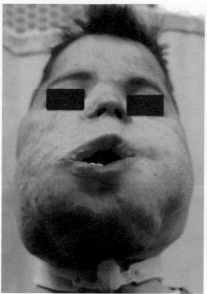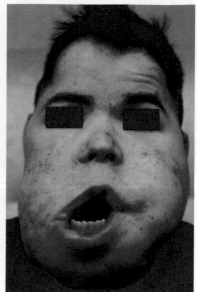

Fig. 1. 16 year old boy with a lymphangioma.

mandible (5.8%), and brain (4.3%).[12] They typically present as a rapidly expanding blueish mass. Despite their aggressive behavior (rapid growth, concomitant destruction of bone, and displacement of adjacent developing teeth), they are mostly benign. A tissue biopsy is necessary to correctly diagnose these lesions and rule out malignancy. A urine test is also helpful because there tends to be high levels of vanillylmandelic acid in urine with melanotic tumors.[2]

Wide local excision is the treatment of choice, with most surgeons advocating the inclusion of a 5-mm margin. Recurrence has been reported in 10% to 20% of cases with adequate resection margins, but can reach up to 45% without wide local excision.[2,3,12]

AGE 2 YEARS AND OLDER
Fibroma

Fibroma is the most common soft tissue lesion in the oral cavity. It is mostly reactive, secondary to irritation or trauma, and histologically appears as a hyperplastic variant of normal tissue. Fibromas can occur anywhere in the mouth that may be easily traumatized, usually by the teeth, such as the buccal and labial mucosa, tongue, and gingiva. They are usually asymptomatic lesions that appear similar in color to the normal mucosa, are well-circumscribed, and generally less than 1 cm in size. Most are sessile, but some are pedunculated. They can occur in any age group. Histologically they demonstrate a nodular mass of fibrous

connective tissue stroma covered by stratified squamous epithelium. The lesion is not encapsulated, and the tissue itself generally blends into the surrounding normal tissue.

Treatment is simple surgical excision, which in most cases can be performed under local anesthesia unless the child exhibits behavioral issues. Recurrence is extremely rare.[2,13–15]

Pyogenic Granuloma, Peripheral Giant Cell Granuloma, Peripheral Ossifying Fibroma

The next most common pathologic lesions seen in the pediatric population are the 3 Ps: pyogenic granuloma, peripheral giant cell granuloma, and peripheral ossifying fibroma. The 3 Ps can appear clinically similar and should be included in the same differential diagnosis, and ultimately require excisional biopsy for diagnosis; however, there can be subtle noted differences between these 3 lesions.

The pyogenic granuloma is a misnomer. It does not, in fact, exhibit granulomatous features, but instead is believed to be a hyperplastic tissue response to local irritation or trauma. It is generally described as a smooth or lobulated mass. The surface is bright red in color with a vascular appearance; however, it can range from pink to red to purple depending on how long the lesion has been present. Typically, pyogenic granuloma presents as a painless, slow-growing mass that can range from a few millimeters in size to several centimeters. They are extremely friable and bleed easily, which is generally responsible for the patient's chief complaint.

Pyogenic granulomas can develop at any age, however, they are most common in children and young adults, with a female predilection. Seventy-five percent of cases present on gingival tissue, likely a result of poor oral hygiene. The lips, tongue, and buccal mucosa are also sites where they develop, and frequently there is a history of trauma to the area. These lesions are more common on the anterior, facial, and maxillary gingival regions, and may extend between teeth (**Fig. 2**).

Histologically, pyogenic granulomas are highly vascular and appear similar to granulation tissue. There are many endothelium-lined channels with red blood cells, and there is usually a mixed inflammatory cell infiltrate consisting of neutrophils, plasma cells, and lymphocytes (**Fig. 3**). Treatment of this lesion in children is full thickness surgical excision. Most of the time this is a curative treatment, however, the lesion can recur and may require re-excision.[2,15–19]

Peripheral giant cell granuloma, or giant cell epulis, is another lesion that is misrepresented in its name and is also reactive, likely caused by local irritation or trauma. The peripheral giant cell granuloma is believed to be the counterpart of the central giant cell granuloma because of their histologic resemblance. The peripheral giant cell granuloma appears exclusively on the anterior or posterior regions of the gingiva or edentulous ridge as a purple-blue nodule. It is more frequently found in the mandible than the maxilla. Most lesions are smaller than 2 cm in diameter and can be sessile, pedunculated, or ulcerated. These lesions can develop at almost any age, usually ranging from the first to the sixth decades of life, with a mean age of 30 to 40 years. Histopathologically, this granuloma appears as a collection of multinucleated giant cells, with a background of ovoid and spindle-shaped mesenchymal cells. Also, deposits of hemosiderin pigment are usually found, often at the periphery of the specimen, as a result of local hemorrhage. Treatment of peripheral giant cell granuloma is full thickness surgical excision, with treatment of the underlying irritant, whether from calculus or local trauma. Ten percent of lesions recur and require local re-excision.[2,14–19]

The peripheral ossifying fibroma is another gingival lesion that is considered to be reactive, with an unknown pathogenesis. It has been hypothesized that some are initially pyogenic granulomas that undergo transformation and calcification. The peripheral ossifying fibroma is usually found in teenagers and young adults (age range from 10 to 19 years) with a female predilection. They are derived from the periodontal ligament, and appear as a pale, nodular growth, usually on the interdental papilla. Peripheral ossifying fibromas occur exclusively on gingival tissue, and most frequently are found in the maxillary arch at the incisor-cuspid region. Most are less than 2 cm in size, however, they may be larger in some cases.

Histologically, there is fibrous proliferation with mineralized product ranging from bone, cementum-like material, or dystrophic calcifications, or a combination of all 3. The standard treatment modality for these lesions is full thickness surgical excision, with a search for an underlying irritant (eg, calculus). If the mass is not excised to include periosteum, there is a higher rate of recurrence. Overall, however, there is an 8% to 16% recurrence rate.[2,15–17,19,20]

Parulis

A parulis is the soft tissue manifestation of a necrotic tooth. Usually these teeth have been chronically infected, and the infection has chosen the path of least resistance through the root apex, buccal cortical bone, and finally through the gingival tissue. They can occur in any age group. On clinical appearance, usually one can express purulence through the center of the parulis or sinus tract. Surrounding the parulis opening is mildly swollen, erythematous, raised gingival tissue, usually no larger than 3 to 4 mm in diameter. One way to confirm that this growth is a parulis, and diagnose from which tooth it originates, is by passing a gutta-percha point through the parulis opening until slight resistance is encountered, and then obtaining a periapical radiograph. On the radiograph, the gutta-percha point will track

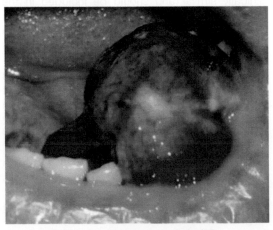

Fig. 2. Left mandibular pyogenic granuloma.

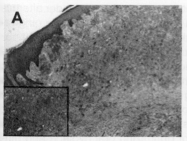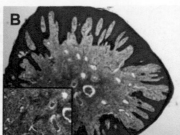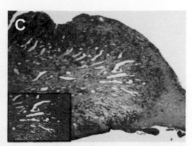

Fig. 3. Photomicrographs differentiating between the 3 most common gingival lesions. (*A*) Peripheral giant cell granuloma, 4× and 10× power, showing multinucleated giant cells with ovoid and spindle-shaped mesenchymal cells in the background. (*B*) Peripheral ossifying fibroma, 4× and 10× power, showing central bone formation. (*C*) Pyogenic granuloma, 4× and 10× power, showing small and large endothelium-lined channels filled with red blood cells.

to the root apex that is the source of infection. Treatment involves finding the source of infection and targeting therapy. Typically, the source requires either an endodontic procedure, or extraction depending on the restorability of the tooth. Antibiotics are normally reserved for use in immunocompromised patients, because immunocompetent hosts tend to respond well to targeted procedures. If necessary, antibiotics are recommended, and include the penicillins, and, if allergic, clindamycin.[2]

Eruption Cyst/Eruption Hematoma

Eruption cysts or eruption hematomas are loosely considered the soft tissue equivalent of dentigerous cysts. They are soft tissue swellings that occur from the separation of the follicle from an erupting tooth, most frequently the deciduous mandibular central or maxillary incisors, and first permanent molars. Clinically, they appear on the alveolar crest superior to an erupting tooth as a soft translucent bubble. If traumatized, they can appear bluish-purple, and may be considered more of an eruption hematoma (**Fig. 4**). Diagnosis is clinical, and treatment is usually not necessary because most teeth will erupt through the cyst and effectively treat the lesion. However, if the cyst persists, becomes secondarily infected, or the tooth does not erupt during the usual time period, the cyst can be surgically unroofed, or marsupialized, to facilitate tooth eruption and cyst drainage.[2–4]

Mucocele

Mucoceles are another type of soft tissue swelling found in the pediatric population. They are often caused by local trauma or irritation, however, the cause is not always easily identified. A patient usually complains of a small painless swelling in the oral cavity that has been present for several weeks or has regressed and recurred on multiple occasions. Mucoceles most frequently occur on the lower lip (about 81% of the time) but can also be found on the floor of mouth, ventral tongue, buccal mucosa, palate, and retromolar trigone (in the location of any minor salivary glands that are found throughout the oral cavity).[21] Clinically, they appear as small, well-circumscribed, translucent soft swellings in the common anatomic areas mentioned earlier (**Fig. 5**). The swelling is secondary to the rupture of small minor salivary glands and subsequent spillage of mucin into the adjacent submucosa. Treatment of a mucocele usually includes excisional biopsy, because only some mucoceles resolve spontaneously. Surgical excision includes removing the affected salivary gland and any associated adjacent minor salivary glands. If a mucocele recurs after surgical treatment, it usually needs to be re-excised, along with additional adjacent minor salivary glands that were likely left behind during the first excision procedure.[2,21,22]

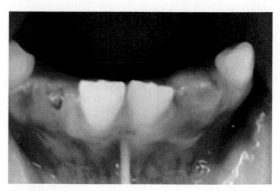

Fig. 4. Eruption cyst associated with an erupting permanent left mandibular lateral incisor. The blueish-purple color indicates an eruption hematoma likely secondary to trauma. (*Courtesy of* Joan Phelan, DDS, New York.)

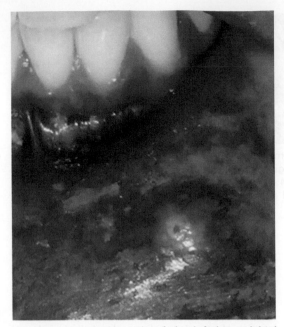

Fig. 5. Recurrent mucocele of the left lower labial mucosa.

Gingival Hyperplasia

Gingival hyperplasia refers literally to the swelling or overgrowth of gingival tissues in localized or generalized regions. There are many different causes for gingival enlargement including response to local inflammation, medications, spongiotic or leukemic infiltrates, mouth breathing, or an idiopathic cause. The key to management is to correctly diagnose and identify the underlying cause in order to target treatment appropriately. In cases where local inflammation is the cause of the gingival hyperplasia, this usually manifests as localized or generalized gingivitis, and the irritating factors must be addressed. Usually, this involves optimizing and maintaining good oral hygiene.

The most common medications that cause gingival hyperplasia include phenytoin (50% develop hyperplasia), cyclosporine (25% develop hyperplasia), and calcium channel blockers (25% develop hyperplasia).[2] The degree of enlargement seems to correspond to oral hygiene and overall susceptibility of the patient. Development of gingival hyperplasia appears within the first 1 to 3 months of drug use, and begins in the interdental papilla, expanding slowly over the buccal surfaces of the teeth. It does not usually occur in edentulous areas. In a patient with good oral hygiene, the tissue will appear as normal gingiva, pink and soft, but overgrown. In a patient with poor oral hygiene, and resultant increased inflammation, the tissue will appear red, friable, and overgrown. The first

line of treatment, if possible, is to consider alternative medication if this is the cause of the gingival hyperplasia. If the patient responds to discontinuance of the causative medication, regression of the hyperplastic tissue will be obvious in 6 to 12 months from the date of drug discontinuation. However, drug discontinuation or switching to another class of medications is not an option in certain circumstances, and the treatment target becomes that of optimizing oral hygiene and ultimately surgical excision of excess tissue, if necessary. Recurrence does occur especially in patients with poor oral hygiene, and may be apparent as soon as 3 months after surgical excision. Usually, however, tissue regrowth is not seen for at least 12 months.[2,3,17]

A less common type of gingival hyperplasia that has recently been distinguished in the literature is localized juvenile spongiotic gingival hyperplasia (**Fig. 6**). This hyperplastic lesion is usually solitary and involves the attached gingiva overlying a tooth root in the anterior maxilla. It has a predilection for female preteens or early adolescents. Clinical appearance consists of a small semilunar erythematous lesion that is easily friable. Histology differs from that of other gingival hyperplasia in that it includes spongiosis and neutrophilic exocytosis. It has been hypothesized that the cause is local foreign body inflammation, and thus treatment involves improvement in oral hygiene. However, it also seems that this gingival hyperplasia might be a self-limiting condition that resolves over time spontaneously without treatment.[23]

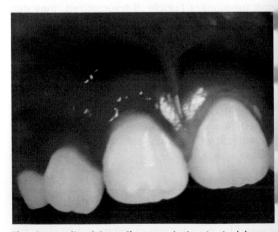

Fig. 6. Localized juvenile spongiotic gingival hyperplasia characterized by a smooth erythematous lesion in the keratinized gingiva superior to tooth 8. (*Courtesy of* Joan Phelan, DDS, New York.)

Aphthous Ulcer

Recurrent aphthous stomatitis, also known as a canker sore, is the most common inflammatory ulcerative process diagnosed in the North American population. It usually first occurs in childhood with 80% noting their first ulceration before the age of 30 years. The exact cause is unknown, however, aphthous ulcers have been directly linked to family history (when both parents are affected the offspring have a 90% chance of developing aphthous stomatitis), food hypersensitivities, trauma, smoking, stress, hormonal states, and infectious or immunologic factors.[2] All these factors, either independently or clustered together, result in the formation of these ulcers by primary immunodysregulation, a decrease in the mucosal barrier, and an increase in antigenic exposure. These aphthous ulcers appear almost exclusively on nonkeratinized tissue. Initially, they appear as focal erythematous lesions that develop into a well-circumscribed, yellow-white, fibrin membrane surrounded by an erythematous halo (**Fig. 7**). Minor ulcers are usually between 3 and 10 mm in diameter, and major ulcers can be 1 to 3 cm in diameter. There is also a herpetiform variant that resembles herpes simplex virus (HSV) infections, however, actually represent only many small, clustered aphthous ulcers.

These ulcers do resolve on their own within 2 to 4 weeks, however, they can be exquisitely painful. Treatment is palliative and includes topical corticosteroids. It is of utmost importance to ascertain a comprehensive medical history because aphthous ulcers may be a sign of an underlying immunodeficiency that may require systemic treatment. These immunodeficiency states include Behçet disease, mouth and genital ulcers with inflamed cartilage (MAGIC) syndrome, cyclic neutropenia, periodic fever with aphthae pharyngitis and adenitis (PFAPA) syndrome, Sweet syndrome, and various nutritional deficiencies (iron, folate, zinc, vitamins B1, B2, B6, B12), with or without underlying gastrointestinal disorders.[24]

Ultimately, clinical diagnosis seems to be the gold standard but tissue biopsy of aphthous lesions can be useful in ruling out other differential diagnoses.[2]

Herpes Simplex Virus

Acute herpetic gingivostomatitis is the most common pattern of HSV-1 infection seen in the pediatric population. It manifests itself in many different ways and is therefore not always diagnosed properly. Most cases present between the ages of 6 months and 5 years and can show symptoms similar to that of a standard flu episode, including cervical lymphadenopathy, chills, fevers, nausea, and sore mouth lesions. The manifestations may vary from mild to severe. Clinically, the oral lesions first appear on both keratinized and nonkeratinized mucosa as small, clustered, vesicular bullae (**Fig. 8**). Throughout their course, they can develop

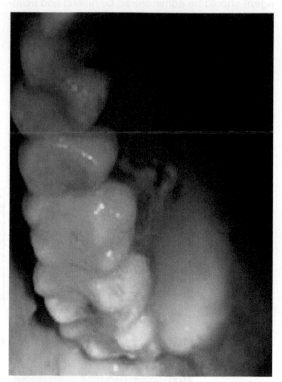

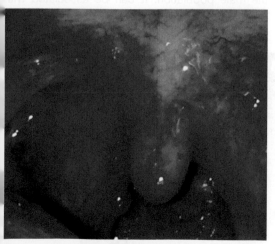

Fig. 7. Minor aphthous ulcer along the right soft palate with a small central area of yellow fibrin with surrounding erythematous halo.

Fig. 8. Primary herpetic gingivostomatitis noted by ulceration and diffuse erythema along the keratinized palatal gingiva of the right maxilla.

into painful widespread ulcerations. Gingival tissues also become enlarged and erythematous.[2,3]

Recurrent HSV infections occur either at the primary infection site or at adjacent areas associated with the involved nerve ganglion, but usually on keratinizing mucosa. The most common site is the lower lip. The patient typically experiences prodromal symptoms at the site (eg, tingling) which then develops into clustered vesicular bullae. These vesicles burst within 2 to 3 days and heal entirely within 1 to 2 weeks. A less common presentation of HSV-1 is infection on the fingers or thumb; an area that can be easily self-inoculated by a child. This is also known as a herpetic whitlow. Diagnosis can usually be made by clinical presentation, however, laboratory tests are suggested for confirmation. These ancillary tests include swabs or smears of the vesicular fluid, tissue biopsy, and collection of blood serum.

HSV infections can be treated in a palliative fashion, however, they can also be preemptively treated with antiviral medications to lessen the magnitude of the outbreak (**Fig. 9**). In primary herpetic gingivostomatitis, acyclovir suspension is a good option for the pediatric population. When treatment is started during the first 3 symptomatic days, resolution is expedited, with decreased pain and other symptoms. The antiviral agent should be administered by rinsing and swallowing (15 mg/kg) 5 times per day for 5 days. In addition, topical spray with 0.5% or 1.0% dyclonine hydrochloride also helps alleviate the pain associated with the lesions. Viscous lidocaine and topical benzocaine should not be used in the pediatric population because it is difficult to titrate the amount of anesthetic that is absorbed, and there have been several reports of lidocaine-induced seizures and methemoglobinemia from the use of excess benzocaine.

For recurrent herpes labialis, penciclovir cream, initiated during the prodrome phase, has the most significant effect on reducing the duration of the HSV outbreak. Systemic medications can be used as well (including acyclovir, valacyclovir, and famciclovir); however, in immunocompetent individuals outbreaks occur infrequently during the year and tend to respond well to topical treatment.[2,3]

Macroglossia

Macroglossia is fairly uncommon and presents with hypertrophy of the tongue. It most often is seen in the pediatric population, and can range from mild to severe with symptoms including noisy breathing, drooling, difficulty eating, speech changes, and airway obstruction. Usually macroglossia is caused by a congenital malformation or systemic disease, most frequently from vascular malformations and muscular hypertrophy. It also is a feature in several syndromes including Beckwith-Wiedemann syndrome and Down syndrome.[25] Treatment is based on the severity of the initial presentation. In most cases, surgical treatment is not indicated, and the child may only require supportive treatments, such as speech therapy. In more severe cases, where there is pending airway compromise, reduction glossectomy is indicated.[2,3,25]

Ankyloglossia

Ankyloglossia, also known as a tongue tie, occurs when the lingual frenum of the tongue is much shorter than the average length and causes limited mobility of the tongue (**Fig. 10**). It occurs in 1.7% to 4.4% of neonates, and 4 times more frequently in the male population. It can be associated with some syndromes, but is usually a primary and

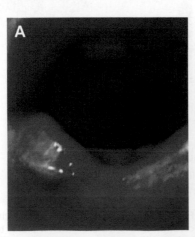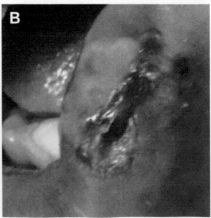

Fig. 9. (*A, B*) Recovering recurrent herpes labialis in 2 different patients.

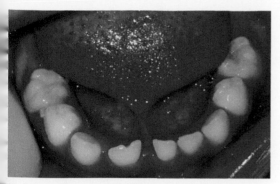

Fig. 10. Ankyloglossia. (*Courtesy of* Aamna Ali, DDS, New York.)

solitary abnormality.[26] Most often, patients can compensate for this limited tongue mobility, but in others, where it impedes mastication or speech, surgical intervention is indicated. The release of the tongue is simply performed by a frenotomy or frenuloplasty procedure and recurrence is minimal when performed appropriately.[2,3]

Soft Tissue Anesthesia Trauma

As mentioned earlier, most pathology in the pediatric population is iatrogenic, secondary to trauma or irritation. One of the most disfiguring pathologies is actually trauma from lip biting after local anesthesia (**Fig. 11**). If not carefully watched or instructed, children will gnaw on whatever soft tissue is anesthetized. A day or two after a procedure, they can present with a swollen, erythroleukoplakic, friable mass, with diffuse fibrin deposits. The diagnosis is clinical and based on a

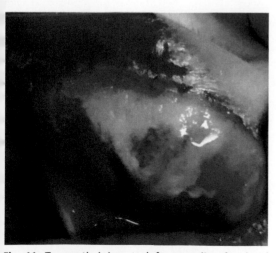

Fig. 11. Traumatic injury to left upper lip after local anesthesia. (*Courtesy of* Bryan Hinkle, DDS, New York.)

thorough history of previous dental treatment. Treatment is palliative.

REFERENCES

1. Jones AV, Franklin CD. An analysis of oral and maxillofacial pathology found in children over a 30-year period. Int J Paediatr Dent 2006;16(1):19–30.
2. Neville BW, Damm DD, Allen CM, et al. Oral and maxillofacial pathology. 3rd edition. St Louis (MO): Saunders Elsevier; 2009.
3. Aldred MJ, Cameron AC. Pediatric oral medicine and pathology. In: Nowak A, Casamassimo P, editors. Handbook of pediatric dentistry. 3rd edition. Philadelphia: Mosby Elsevier; 2008. p. 192–216.
4. Hays P. Hamartomas, eruption cysts, natal tooth, and Epstein pearls in a newborn. J Dent Child 2000;67:365–8.
5. Kilcline C, Frieden IJ. Infantile hemangiomas: how common are they? A systematic review of the medical literature. Pediatr Dermatol 2008;25:168–73.
6. Chen ZG, Zheng JW, Yuan ML, et al. A novel topical nano-propranolol for treatment of infantile hemangiomas. Nanomedicine 2015;11:1109–15.
7. Hoff SR, Rastatter JC, Richter GT. Head and neck vascular lesions. Otolaryngol Clin North Am 2015;48:29–45.
8. Buckmiller L, Richter G, Suen J. Diagnosis and management of hemangiomas and vascular malformations of the head and neck. Oral Dis 2010;16(5):405–18.
9. Aparna HG, Jayanth BS, Shashidara R, et al. Congenital epulis in a newborn: a case report, immunoprofiling and review of the literature. Ethiop J Health Sci 2014;24:359–62.
10. Ritwik P, Brannon RB, Musselman RJ. Spontaneous regression of congenital epulis: a case report and review of the literature. J Med Case Rep 2010;4:331.
11. Anderson PJ, Kirkland P, Schafler K, et al. Congenital gingival granular cell tumour. J R Soc Med 1996;89:53–4.
12. Gupta R, Kumar S, Saxena S. Melanotic neuroectodermal tumor of infancy: review of literature, report of a case and follow up at 7 years. J Plast Reconstr Aesthet Surg 2015;68:53–4.
13. Shapira M, Akrish S. A 6-year-old girl with a lesion on the tongue. Pediatr Ann 2011;40:71–4.
14. Magnusson BC, Rasmusson LG. The giant cell fibroma – A review of 103 cases with immunohistochemical findings. Acta Odontol Scand 1995;53:293–6.
15. Shah KS, Le MC, Carpenter WM. Retrospective review of pediatric oral lesions from a dental school biopsy service. Pediatr Dent 2009;31:14–9.
16. Kamath K, Vidya M, Anand P. Biopsied lesions of the gingiva in a southern Indian population – a retrospective study. Oral Health Prev Dent 2013;11:71–9.

17. Anneroth G, Sigurdson A. Hyperplastic lesions of the gingiva and alveolar mucosa – a study of 175 cases. Acta Odontol Scand 1983;41:75–86.

18. Krishnapillai R, Punnoose K, Angadi PV, et al. Oral pyogenic granuloma – a review of 215 cases in a south Indian teaching hospital, Karnataka, over a period of 20 years. Oral Maxillofac Surg 2012;16:305–9.

19. Buchner A, Scnaiderman-Shapiro A, Vered M. Pediatric localized reactive gingival lesions: a retrospective study from Israel. Pediatr Dent 2010;32:486–92.

20. Moon WJ, Choi SY, Chung EC, et al. Peripheral ossifying fibroma in the oral cavity: CT and MR findings. Dentomaxillofac Radiol 2007;36:180–2.

21. Chi A, Lampbert P, Richardson M, et al. Oral mucoceles: a clinicopathologic review of 1824 cases including unusual variants. J Oral Maxillofac Surg 2011;69:1086–93.

22. Baurmash HD. Mucoceles and ranulas. J Oral Maxillofac Surg 2003;61:369–78.

23. Solomon LW, Trahan WR, Snow J. Localized juvenile spongiotic gingival hyperplasia: a report of 3 cases. Pediatr Dent 2013;35:360–3.

24. Gurkan A, Ozlu SG, Altiaylik-Ozer P, et al. Recurrent aphthous stomatitis in childhood and adolescence: a single-center experience. Pediatr Dermatol 2015;32:476–80.

25. Costa SA, Brinhole MCP, da Silva RA, et al. Surgical treatment of congenital true macroglossia. Case Rep Dent 2013;2013:489194.

26. Chandrashekar L, Kashinath KR, Suhas S. Labial ankyloglossia associated with oligodontia: a case report. J Dent (Tehran) 2014;11:481–4.

Pediatric Head and Neck Malignancies

Mohammed Qaisi, DMD, MD[a,b,*], Issam Eid, MD[b]

KEYWORDS

- Pediatric malignancies • Pediatric tumors • Pediatric head and neck malignancies
- Pediatric head and neck tumors • Pediatric sarcomas • Pediatric carcinoma

KEY POINTS

- Pediatric head and neck malignancies are rare, and therefore there is a lack of high-level evidence to guide treatment.
- Pediatric head and neck malignancies are often treated with multimodality treatment. One must be cognizant of the potential side effects on young growing patients.
- In surgical diseases, obtaining clear surgical margins seems to be the single most important prognostic factor in improving survival.

Head and neck (H&N) malignancies are rare in pediatric patients, and represent 12% of all pediatric malignancies.[1] The incidence of these H&N tumors is 1.49 cases per 1,000,000 person-years. Despite that, pediatric malignancies account for the second largest cause death in children, after accidental trauma.

Among the most common pediatric H&N malignancies are lymphomas (27%), neural tumors including primitive neurectodermal tumors (PNET; 23%), thyroid malignancies (21%), soft tissue sarcomas (12%), nasopharyngeal carcinoma, skeletal malignancies, and salivary gland malignancies.[2]

Although an exhaustive review of all pediatric H&N malignancies is beyond the scope of this article, the most common and relevant malignancies that affect children are discussed, with the exception of salivary gland malignancies, which are discussed elsewhere in this issue.

LYMPHOMA

Hematogenous malignancies are the most common cancers in children. Of these, acute lymphocytic leukemia is the most common, accounting for about one-third of pediatric malignancies. Lymphomas rank as the most common pediatric cancer.[2] They are divided into Hodgkin lymphoma and non-Hodgkin lymphoma (NHL). There have been significant advances in the treatment of these diseases in the last 30 years and survival has more than doubled, with cure rates for lymphomas approaching 90%.[3]

Hodgkin lymphoma has a bimodal distribution with a peak in adolescence and adulthood. Approximately 1000 new cases present in the pediatric age group annually in the United States. The incidence is 50 per million, and only 5% of tumors occur in children younger than age 10. The pediatric disease has a male preponderance (2:1 male/female ratio) and has been associated with the Epstein-Barr virus.[4] Most of these patients (about 80%) present with asymptomatic cervical adenopathy, without "B" symptoms (fever, night sweats, weight loss), which can be associated with Hodgkin lymphoma and NHL and have prognostic significance (staging).[5] This disease can be broadly divided into two categories: the more common "classical" Hodgkin lymphoma, comprising 90% of cases, and the "lymphocyte-predominant" type of

[a] Department of Oral and Maxillofacial Surgery, University of Mississippi Medical Center, 2500 N. State Street, Jackson, MS 39216, USA; [b] Department of Otolaryngology, University of Mississippi Medical Center, 2500 N. State Street, Jackson, MS 39216, USA
* Corresponding author. Department of Oral and Maxillofacial Surgery, University of Mississippi Medical Center, Jackson, MS 39216.
E-mail address: mqaisi@umc.edu

Oral Maxillofacial Surg Clin N Am 28 (2016) 11–19
http://dx.doi.org/10.1016/j.coms.2015.07.008
1042-3699/16/$ – see front matter © 2016 Elsevier Inc. All rights reserved.

Hodgkin lymphoma. Classical Hodgkin disease is further classified into the following subtypes, in the order of prevalence: nodular sclerosing Hodgkin lymphoma (65%), mixed cellularity Hodgkin lymphoma (22%), and lymphocyte depleted Hodgkin (rare in children).[6] The Ann Arbor staging system is used to stage these tumors according to whether disease is localized, and whether it involves organs on both sides of the diaphragm. Staging work-up should include a computed tomography of the neck, chest, and abdomen. Blood tests that are indicated include a complete blood count with differential, erythrocyte sedimentation rate, renal and hepatic function tests, and alkaline phosphatase. A histopathologic hallmark of this disease is the Reed-Sternberg cells.[4] Treatment is nonsurgical, and is based on risk stratification, and also depends on the stage of the disease. Lymph node biopsy is often needed for diagnosis because fine-needle aspiration (FNA) biopsy often has a low diagnostic yield. Early and low-risk localized disease has been traditionally treated with radiation with acceptable cure rates. Advanced and high-risk disease is treated with a combination of multiagent chemotherapy and radiotherapy.[6] Recent trends in the treatment of Hodgkin disease have shifted toward multimodality therapy to limit the toxicities associated with chemotherapy and radiation therapy.

NHL has a male preponderance with a 2:1 to 3:1 male/female ratio, and it is more common in white persons. Systematic reviews have shown an overall increase in annual incidence of this disease since the mid-1970s with 600 new cases occurring annually in the United States.[7] Unlike the bimodal distribution in Hodgkin disease, NHL has an increasing incidence with age, with only 25% of cases occurring in children younger than age 10.[7] Adult NHL tends to be typically a nodal disease; in contrast, pediatric lymphoma has a propensity for involving extranodal sites. Most cases present in the mediastinum or abdomen, but about 10% of cases present primarily in the H&N. The most commonly involved sites in the H&N include cervical lymph nodes, salivary glands, larynx, sinuses, orbit, and Waldeyer ring.[8] This disease tends to be grow rapidly, and early diagnosis is critical for prompt appropriate treatment. The histopathology of these diseases is widely varied and generally categorized into low, intermediate, and high grade depending on how aggressive the tumor behaves. Most tumors in children are high-grade lesions.[9] The most common NHLs in children are mature B-cell lymphomas, which includes Burkitt lymphoma and diffuse large B-cell lymphomas, followed by lymphoblastic and anaplastic large cell lymphomas.[3]

Diagnosis is established via incisional biopsy and histopathologic analysis of the involved tissue. As in Hodgkin disease, FNA tends to be of limited value. A cervical lymph node excision is the preferred method for diagnosis in cases of cervical adenopathy.[10] Biopsy tissue should be sent fresh (not fixed) for histopathology to facilitate flow cytometry, immunohistochemical staining, and other specialized stains and testing. Surgery is reserved for a diagnostic role, with the mainstay of treatment being multiagent chemotherapy. A CHOP-based regimen (cyclophosphamide, hydroxydaunomycin, vincristine, and prednisone) is most commonly used in these cases. Prognosis depends on the stage, and with recent advances in chemotherapy regimens achieving survival of more than 80% is typical.[3]

RHABDOMYOSARCOMA

Whereas in the adult patient rhabdomyosarcoma accounts for a minority of the pathology of H&N cancers, this malignancy is one of the most common tumors of childhood. It affects about 250 children per year in the United States.[11] It is the third most common soft tissue malignant neoplasm after Wilms tumor and neuroblastoma, accounting for 13% of all pediatric cancers. The H&N is the most common site of rhabdomyoscarcoma, accounting for 35% to 40% of these tumors.

These tumors are bimodal in distribution, and often present in patients younger than 5 years of age and between 10 and 18 years of age.[12] An asymptomatic mass is the most common presenting finding. Within the H&N, the eye is a very common subsite for rhabdomyoscarcoma, followed by the oral cavity (**Fig. 1**) and the pharynx.

Histologically, rhabdomyosarcoma is one of the "small round blue cell" tumors, presenting with sheets of small cells with large prominent nuclei. Rhabdomyosarcoma is divided according to histopathology into three distinct categories: (1) embryonal, (2) alveolar, and (3) pleomorphic. The embryonal type is most common at birth, and the alveolar form peaks in childhood and adolescence.[13] Embryonal is the most common type accounting for 75% of H&N cases, with the botryoid subtype demonstrating a more favorable prognosis.[14] Alveolar rhabdomyosarcoma has a worse prognosis. The 5-year survival rate for the embryonal type is 97% in nonorbital, nonparameningeal cases, whereas the alveolar type has a survival rate of 67%.[15]

Management of these tumors is often multimodal, with chemotherapy playing a key role. The Intergroup Rhabdomyosarcoma Study (IRS I-IV) has established a staging and grouping

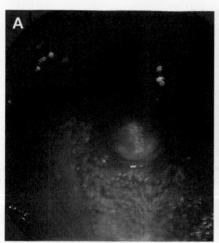
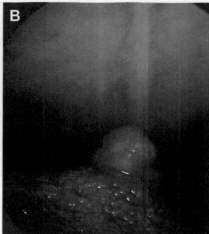

Fig. 1. (*A, B*) Two views of a sessile mass at the base of tongue, with biopsy positive for rhabdomyosarcoma.

system for rhabdomyosarcoma that directs ideal therapy, based on whether the disease is localized or metastatic, and whether or not it is resectable.[16] Group I consists of localized disease that is completely excised with pathologically clear margins. Group II includes patients with gross tumor removal, with residual microscopic disease at margins, or presence of involved regional lymph nodes, or both. Group III is comprised of localized disease, with gross residual disease after incomplete excision or biopsy only. Group IV includes patients with distant metastatic disease at the onset of presentation.

Recently there has been a trend requiring the involvement of surgical management of H&N disease as a definitive therapy.[17] Primary surgical resection with complete excision is recommended for localized disease. Surgery is also indicated for salvage when there is resectable residual local and regional disease.[16] The goal of definitive surgical therapy is to avoid radiation therapy because of the long-term complications and side effects. However, radiation is often necessary for gross residual disease, and in group II patients and higher. The clinically and radiographically negative neck is not generally treated with prophylactic radiotherapy.

Other less common nonrhabdomyosarcoma soft tissue tumors include fibrosarcoma, synovial sarcoma, dermatofibrosarcoma protuberans, malignant fibrous histiocytoma, chondrosarcoma, and liposarcoma.

THYROID CARCINOMA

Thyroid carcinoma is a relatively rare disease of childhood. The annual incidence is 2.4 per 100,000. Although pediatric thyroid carcinomas make up only 2% of all thyroid cancers, the chance of a solitary nodule being cancerous in children is

four times more likely than in adults. A total of 20% of solitary nodules in children are cancerous, compared with only 5% in adult patients.[18] Presentation is usually as a mass in the thyroid region; however, symptoms of dysphonia or odynophagia can also be present. Most cancers are of the papillary variant, and the follicular and anaplastic varieties are rare. There is a female preponderance for thyroid cancer after puberty. Children also have a higher rate of cervical (75%) or pulmonary (5%–20%) metastasis at time of diagnosis, and therefore need to undergo a comprehensive metastatic work-up. Children with multiple endocrine neoplasia types IIA and II B and RET protooncogene mutation frequently develop medullary thyroid carcinoma as part of their disease. It is the most common cause of death in these patients. It leads to early metastasis and is resistant to chemoradiation therapy. Prophylactic total thyroidectomy is advocated in patients with multiple endocrine neoplasia and this RET protooncogene mutation.[19,20] The greatest known risk factor for nonsporadic thyroid cancer is radiation exposure followed by a genetic etiology. FNA is not as well established in the pediatric population as it is in adult patients. When FNA is indeterminate, it may be reasonable to repeat the study in 3 to 6 months, or simply proceed with surgery based on clinical suspicion of the disease. In children younger than 10 years of age, or with a family history of thyroid cancer, prompt surgical resection is advisable without the need for FNA (**Fig. 2**).[2]

NASOPHARYNGEAL CARCINOMA

Nasopharyngeal cancer in childhood is a rare disease. The median age at presentation is 13 years, with male preponderance.[21] This aggressive cancer tends to be diagnosed after presenting as an

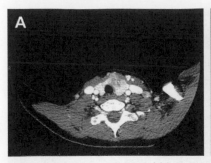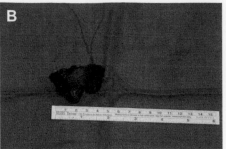

Fig. 2. (*A*) Left thyroid mass in a 9-year-old boy. FNA was positive for papillary thyroid carcinoma. (*B*) Thyroid specimen after total thyroidectomy. (*Courtesy of* Lana Jackson, MD, University of Mississippi Medical Center, Jackson, Mississippi.)

asymptomatic neck mass, often with the use of a lymph node biopsy. Patients may also present with symptoms that mimic the common cold, with nasal obstruction or rhinitis.[2] Nasopharyngeal cancer in children is often associated with an Epstein-Barr viral infection, which generally confers a worse prognosis.[21] The histologic subtype that most frequently presents in children is the World Health Organization type III or undifferentiated variant, as opposed to types I and II, which represent the keratinized and nonkeratinized carcinoma variants, respectively. Treatment usually involves a combination of radiation and chemotherapy.[22] Survival and prognosis is directly related to stage at presentation, with lymph node metastases representing a significant predictor of treatment failure.

OSTEOSARCOMA

Osteosarcoma is the most common pediatric malignancy of bone in the H&N followed by Ewing sarcoma (ES) and chondrosarcoma. It is a rare tumor, overall comprising only 0.5% of all H&N sarcomas in children.[1] Osteosarcoma most frequently occurs in the long bones, with only 10% occurring in the H&N region. The mandible and maxilla are the most commonly involved sites in the H&N.[1–3]

Osteosarcomas of the H&N seem to have a better prognosis than their counterpart in the long bones, with survival rates of 80%.[23,24] The age of onset of H&N cases is one to two decades older than in long bone cases. In the pediatric population, the average age at presentation is around 15 years.[25] Osteosarcomas tend to spread via a hematogenous route, and metastasize to the lungs and other sites. H&N osteosarcomas do not metastasize to distant sites as frequently as long bone cases, with a 17% metastasis in H&N cases versus 80% in long bones.[23]

Osteosarcoma has three histologic subtypes: (1) osteoblastic, (2) chondroblastic, and (3) fibroblastic. The osteoblastic type is the most common variant in long bone cases, which confers a worse prognosis. The most common type in H&N cases is the chondroblastic type. Clinical presentation usually includes jaw swelling, pain, and parasthesia. The classic "sunburst" appearance may be seen on radiographic imaging in about 20% to 40% of cases.

Because of the rarity of this tumor, there is a lack of high-quality data to help guide treatment. In osteosarcoma of the long bones, induction chemotherapy is usually used before surgery. However, in H&N cases there is a lack of data to support this modality over an up-front surgical approach.[24] The single most important prognostic factor seems to be the ability to obtain clear surgical margins. Therefore up-front surgical resection is a reasonable option to avoid delay, and because H&N cases behave more favorably than in the long bones. Postoperative chemotherapy may be used based on the tumor grade and stage. Radiation therapy is usually added to the chemotherapy regimen in cases where surgical margins are involved.

PERIPHERAL PRIMITIVE NEUROECTODERMAL TUMORS

Peripheral PNET (pPNET) is a category of neuroectodermal tumors that falls within the wider umbrella of PNET. PNET also includes tumors that arise from the central nervous system, such as medulloblastoma, and tumors arising from the autonomic system, such as neuroblastoma. As implied by the name, pPNET involve peripheral tissues and nerves, and do not involve the central or autonomic systems.[26]

According to Bataskis and coworkers,[26] pPNET can be further divided, and encompass the following tumors, the first three of which are discussed in this article: malignant pPNET, ES, melanotic neuroectodermal tumors, Askin tumor, ectomesenchymoma, and peripheral medulloepithelioma.

Malignant Peripheral Primitive Neuroectodermal Tumor

Malignant pPNET is a neuroectodermal tumor, and one the rare malignancies that can affect the H&N region. They comprise less than 1% of all sarcomas. They tend to involve the H&N region in 23% to 42% of cases. Most of these tumors tend to occur in children, with a mean age of 15 to 17 years.[27] A review by Nikitakis and colleagues[28] regarding H&N pPNET identified 43 cases between 1965 and 2002, with 63% occurring in the pediatric age group population.

pPNET clinically present as rapidly enlarging and often painful soft tissue masses. The most commonly involved sites in the H&N include the orbit, neck, and parotid glands, but may also involve the maxilla, nasal cavity, sinuses, and skull base.[28,29] The prognosis of malignant pPNET is very poor, with disease-free survival rates of 30% to 45% at 5 years. They have a propensity to metastasize to distant sites, with the most common locations involving the lung, liver, and bone.[30] Orbital pPNET seem to have a more favorable behavior, respond better to treatment, and do not tend to metastasize.

Histologically, malignant pPNET present as small round blue cell tumors, with sheets of small round cells with large prominent nuclei and a high nuclear-to-cytoplasmic ratio. There are numerous tumors that have the same appearance histologically, and the differential diagnosis for small round blue cell tumors includes rhabdomyosarcoma, lymphoma, lymphoblastic leukemia, synovial sarcoma, neuroblastoma, and ES.[26] Malignant pPNET may be differentiated histologically from other small round blue cell tumors by the presence of neural differentiation.

pPNET and ES are thought to be closely related; they are thought to represent two entities along the same spectrum with malignant pPNET showing well-differentiated histology and ES exhibiting the poorly differentiated form. Immunohistochemical staining for MIC-2 (CD99) aids in the diagnosis because it is present in most malignant pPNET and ES, differentiating them from other round blue cell tumors. On a molecular level, malignant pPNET and ES are characterized by translocation between chromosomes 11 and 22, t(11;22)(q24;12), which is present in 85% to 90% of cases.[31]

Treatment modalities include up-front surgery, followed by adjuvant chemoradiation for localized resectable disease.[29] An alternate treatment approach includes the use of induction chemotherapy to help shrink the tumor before resection and decrease the chance of micrometastasis. Chemotherapy usually involves a multiagent high-risk sarcoma protocol. The single most important factor with regards to treatment and improving survival is obtaining clear surgical margins, which may not always be feasible in the H&N, depending on the specific location.

Ewing Sarcoma

ES is the second most common malignancy of bone after osteosarcoma in the pediatric population.[1] ES is one of the PNET tumors and is thought to be closely related to malignant pPNET.

ES is a rare malignancy of children, and makes up 0.05% of all pediatric H&N sarcomas. Only 1% to 7% of ES occur in the H&N region in the pediatric patient age group. The mean age of presentation is 7.5 to 14 years of age.[32] The most commonly involved sites in the H&N include the mandible and skull base.[33]

The clinical presentation usually includes an enlarging mass in the mandible. Orbital lesions are often associated with proptosis, periorbital edema, and decreasing visual acuity.[32] ES may present with distant metastasis at time of initial presentation in 15% to 30% of cases, which greatly affects prognosis. Metastasis at presentation is associated with a 30% 5-year survival, as opposed to a 65% 5-year survival for localized disease.

Similar to malignant pPNET, ES is a small round blue cell tumor histologically that stains with MIC (CD99) and has a translocation between chromosome 11 and 22 in 85% to 90% of cases. These two entities are difficult to differentiate histologically, and malignant pPNET tend to have more neuronal differentiation and neuronal rossettes.[28]

Treatment usually involves a 4- to 6-week course of induction chemotherapy followed by surgical resection, even for localized disease.[34] This therapy is then followed by postoperative chemotherapy. Radiotherapy is reserved for use in combination with chemotherapy in cases of unresectable tumors, or in the presence of residual disease or positive margins. Orbital tumors are usually treated with chemoradiation therapy, and surgery is often avoided because of the associated morbidity. The IESS-II study demonstrated a 68% response rate in patients receiving a high-dose regimen of vincristine, adriamycin, and cyclophosphamide.

Malignant Melanotic Neuroectodermal Tumor of Infancy

Melanotic neuroectodermal tumor of infancy (MNTI) is one of the pPNETs.[26] It is thought to be derived from a neural crest origin and differs from other PNETs in being a biphasic tumor with two cell populations. It is comprised of polygonal epithelioid cells resembling melanocytes, and small round blue cells, or neuroblast-like cells.[35] Some of these tumors secrete vanillylmandelic acid, which can be measured in the urine, and this supports the theory regarding its neurectodermal origin.[36] Clinically they present as a painless, pigmented, rapidly growing, expansile mass, most often in the maxilla. Although they are considered benign tumors, MNTI tend to be aggressive with frequent recurrences between 20% and 60%,[36,37] with most recurrences occurring within 6 months.[35] MNTI occurs in the H&N in 93% of cases. The most commonly involved sites are the maxilla (75%), mandible (5.8%), calvarium (10.8%), and brain. These tumors usually tend to occur within the first year of life.

A malignant variant of this entity exists and comprises roughly 6.5% of all MNTI.[36] These are rare tumors, with only 24 malignant cases reported between 1918 and 2004.[35] The most commonly involved sites in the malignant type include the brain and calvarium. The maxilla and mandible (**Fig. 3**) are only involved in 25% of cases. These tumors display an increased number of mitotic figures, with the small round blue cell component comprising the more aggressive component of the biphasic tumor. These tumors have a tendency to metastasize to regional lymph nodes, brain, liver, pleura, bone marrow, and pelvis. The prognosis is poor, with more than 65% of patients succumbing to their disease within the first 2 years of life.[38]

Treatment of these malignant MNTI often involves multimodality therapy. Surgery with clear margins, when feasible, seems to be the most important prognostic factor. Multidrug chemotherapeutic regimens are often used in the preoperative or postoperative setting.[39] Radiation therapy can be added in the presence of positive margins or inoperable disease.

LANGERHAN CELL HISTOCYTOSIS (HISTOCYTOSIS X)

Langerhan cell histocytosis (LCH) is considered a myeloid neoplasm characterized by an abnormal proliferation of a distinct type of histiocytes known as Langerhan cells (LC). These cells are dendritic cells and are normally found in the epidermis, bone marrow, and lymph nodes. They typically play a role in immunity and function as antigen-presenting cells.

LCH typically tends to involve the pediatric population. Previously, it was thought that there were three distinct types that were grouped under this category; however, it is now believed that these three types are, in fact, one entity, and represent different phases along a continuum, based on the level of systemic involvement and the acuteness of the disease.[40]

Eosinophilic granuloma represents the solitary type of LCH, with one or more lytic bone lesions without visceral involvement. Hand-Schüller-Christian disease is considered the chronic disseminated type and involves bone, skin, and viscera. It is characterized by the triad of bone lesions, exophthalmos, and polyuria. Letterer-Siwe disease occurs predominantly in infants and represents the acute disseminated type. It is a fulminant disease with multiorgan involvement, and presents with hepatosplenomegaly, lymphadenopathy, bone lesions, prominent skin involvement, and

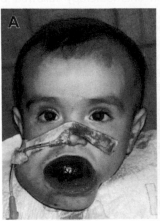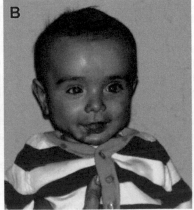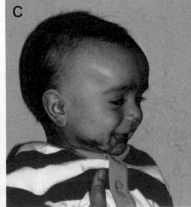

Fig. 3. (*A*) A 6-month-old boy with mandibular malignant melanotic neuroectodermal tumor of infancy. (*B, C*) Two views of patient 3 weeks following tumor resection and neck dissection because of nodal disease. Treatment included chemotherapy, and at 5 years of age the patient is disease-free. (*Courtesy of* Daniel Petrisor, DMD, MD, FACS, Oregon Health Science University School of Dentistry, Portland, Oregon and G.E. Ghali, DDS, MD, FACS, Louisiana State University Health Sciences Center, Shreveport, LA.)

pancytopenia. Cutaneous symptoms are often the initial presentation in these syndromes, and often appear in the form of seborrheic dermatitis-like lesions on the face, scalp, and other sites.[41] Skin biopsies are usually required to confirm the diagnosis.

The annual incidence of LCH is four to eight cases per million in children and one to two per million in adults. Any bone can be involved in LCH, with the calvarium as the most common site. The mandible may also be involved, and may be the first manifestation of a more generalized disease.[42] Lesions in the mandible can mimic periodontial disease with bleeding on probing, tooth mobility, and severe alveolar bone loss. Panoramic radiograph may show the classic "teeth floating in air" appearance.[42] Treatment of self-limited, solitary lesions of the mandible usually includes enucleation and curettage, and the prognosis is excellent. In contrast, acute LCH with multiorgan systemic involvement requires treatment with chemotherapy, with the gold standard of a prednisone/vinblastine combination used alone, or in conjunction with other agents.[43] Because solitary and systemic forms have the same appearance histologically, it is important that patients obtain a thorough work-up because of treatment implications.

Histologically LCH lesions demonstrate an accumulation of LC in an infiltrate of eosinophils, lymphocytes, macrophages, and multinucleated giant cells.[44] LC contain intracytoplasmic Birbeck granules, which are specific to LCH and can aid in the diagnosis. Diagnosis can also be confirmed by immunohistochemical staining for S-100, CD1, and CD207 (Langerin).[40]

In the past, LCH was thought to represent an aberrant and hyperactive immune response. However, more recent literature has validated that LCH is truly a neoplastic process of the myeloid system with clonal accumulations of LC.[45] Most recently, a mutation in the BRAF gene (BRAF V600E) has been identified that supports this hypothesis and is present in 40% to 60% of LCH cases.[40] This gene can be used as target for treatment, and may be used to assess efficacy of treatment because it can be detected in the serum. These recent advances in the understanding of the molecular aspect of LCH will have positive implications on treatment and open the way for targeted therapy.

AMELOBLASTIC CARCINOMA

According to the World Health Organization, ameloblastic carcinoma (AC) is defined as a tumor that demonstrates the morphologic features of ameloblastoma with atypia, including increased mitotic figures and plemorphism, regardless of the presence or absence of metastasis.[46] AC is classified as primary or secondary types depending on whether they arise de novo or secondarily from an ameloblastoma.

AC is a rare malignancy, especially in children. In a review of AC cases in pediatric patients between 1932 and 2012, only 18 cases were identified.[46] The mean age was 12.6 years (range, 4–17 years), and all were of the primary AC type.

Clinically, these tumors tend to involve the mandible and the maxilla with a predilection for the mandible in a ratio of 1:1 to 3:1 over the maxilla. The overall mean age at diagnosis is 30 years. AC is locally aggressive and can cause bony destruction, pain, ulceration, and parasthesia. Metastases occurs via hematogenous spread to a greater extent, and via lymphatics; thus, regional lymph nodes may be involved, and a prophylactic neck dissection is advocated in AC cases.[47] The most common site of distant metastasis is the lungs. Other sites include the brain, liver, bone, and kidneys. AC requires long-term surveillance because of the possibility of late recurrence many years after surgical resection.[46] The prognosis for this tumor is poor, and depends largely on the presence of distant metastasis and local control and the ability to obtain clear surgical margins.[47]

In the absence of distant metastasis, surgical resection of the involved area and neck dissection seem to be clinically indicated. The role of radiation and chemotherapy is unclear, and is often reserved for unresectable tumors or for palliative therapy. Radiotherapy may be used for close surgical margins, or the presence of adverse features, such as perineural invasion.

Malignant ameloblastoma or metastasizing ameloblastoma is a separate entity not to be confused with AC. Metastasizing ameloblastoma is a benign ameloblastoma that develops distant metastasis, most frequently in the lungs, with the same benign histology as the primary tumor.[48] Metastasis usually occurs late, occurring on average 9 to 18 years after the initial primary, and therefore the diagnosis is seldom made in pediatric patients.[48] The primary site usually develops multiple recurrences requiring multiple operations, often because of undertreatment at the initial surgery. The prognosis of metastasizing ameloblastoma is excellent despite the presence of metastasis because of the benign nature of the disease. Metastasis may be treated with local excision when feasible.[49]

SUMMARY

Pediatric H&N malignancies are rare and comprise 12% of all malignancies in children. A comprehensive, but not all-inclusive, review of pediatric H&N malignancies is presented in this article. Many of these tumors, depending on the stage, site, and histology, require multimodality treatment. Morbid mutilating surgery with little survival benefit should be avoided. Postoperative radiation therapy can have life-long side effects especially in the growing patient (discussed elsewhere in this issue).

REFERENCES

1. Albright JT, Topham AK, Reilly JS. Pediatric head and neck malignancies: US incidence and trends over 2 decades. Arch Otolaryngol Head Neck Surg 2002;128(6):655–9.
2. Chadha NK, Forte V. Pediatric head and neck malignancies. Curr Opin Otolaryngol Head Neck Surg 2009;17(6):471–6.
3. Gross TG, Termuhlen AM. Pediatric non-Hodgkin's lymphoma. Curr Oncol Rep 2007;9(6):459–65.
4. Weiner MA, Leventhal BG, Marcus R, et al. Intensive chemotherapy and low-dose radiotherapy for the treatment of advanced-stage Hodgkin's disease in pediatric patients: a Pediatric Oncology Group study. J Clin Oncol 1991;9(9):1591–8.
5. Smith RS, Chen Q, Hudson MM, et al. Prognostic factors for children with Hodgkin's disease treated with combined-modality therapy. J Clin Oncol 2003;21(10):2026–33.
6. Olson MR, Donaldson SS. Treatment of pediatric Hodgkin lymphoma. Curr Treat Options Oncol 2008;9(1):81–94.
7. O'Leary M, Sheaffer B, Keller F, et al. Lymphomas and reticuloendothelial neoplasms. In: Bleyer A, O'Leary M, Barr R, et al, editors. Cancer epidemiology in older adolescents and young adults 15 to 29 years of age, including SEER incidence and survival: 1975-2000. Bethesda (MD): National Cancer Institute 2006; p. 25–38.
8. Harley EH. Asymmetric tonsil size in children. Arch Otolaryngol Head Neck Surg 2002;128(7):767–9.
9. Sandlund JT, Downing JR, Crist WM. Non-Hodgkin's lymphoma in childhood. N Engl J Med 1996;334(19):1238–48.
10. Morris-Stiff G, Cheang P, Key S, et al. Does the surgeon still have a role to play in the diagnosis and management of lymphomas? World J Surg Oncol 2008;6:13.
11. Simon JH, Paulino AC, Smith RB, et al. Prognostic factors in head and neck rhabdomyosarcoma. Head Neck 2002;24(5):468–73.
12. Miller RW, Young JL, Novakovic B. Childhood cancer. Cancer 1995;75(1 Suppl):395–405.
13. Toro JR, Travis LB, Wu HJ, et al. Incidence patterns of soft tissue sarcomas, regardless of primary site, in the surveillance, epidemiology and end results

program, 1978-2001: an analysis of 26,758 cases. Int J Cancer 2006;119(12):2922–30.
14. Leaphart C, Rodeberg D. Pediatric surgical oncology: management of rhabdomyosarcoma. Surg Oncol 2007;16(3):173–85.
15. Pappo AS, Meza JL, Donaldson SS, et al. Treatment of localized nonorbital, nonparameningeal head and neck rhabdomyosarcoma: lessons learned from intergroup rhabdomyosarcoma studies III and IV. J Clin Oncol 2003;21(4):638–45.
16. Gillespie MB, Marshall DT, Day TA, et al. Pediatric rhabdomyosarcoma of the head and neck. Curr Treat Options Oncol 2006;7(1):13–22.
17. Daya H, Chan HS, Sirkin W, et al. Pediatric rhabdomyosarcoma of the head and neck: is there a place for surgical management? Arch Otolaryngol Head Neck Surg 2000;126(4):468–72.
18. Dinauer CA, Breuer C, Rivkees SA. Differentiated thyroid cancer in children: diagnosis and management. Curr Opin Oncol 2008;20(1):59–65.
19. Sanso GE, Domene HM, Garcia R, et al. Very early detection of RET proto-oncogene mutation is crucial for preventive thyroidectomy in multiple endocrine neoplasia type 2 children: presence of C-cell malignant disease in asymptomatic carriers. Cancer 2002;94(2):323–30.
20. Moore SW, Appfelstaedt J, Zaahl MG. Familial medullary carcinoma prevention, risk evaluation, and RET in children of families with MEN2. J Pediatr Surg 2007;42(2):326–32.
21. Ayan I, Kaytan E, Ayan N. Childhood nasopharyngeal carcinoma: from biology to treatment. Lancet Oncol 2003;4(1):13–21.
22. Ayan I, Altun M. Nasopharyngeal carcinoma in children: retrospective review of 50 patients. Int J Radiat Oncol Biol Phys 1996;35(3):485–92.
23. Patel SG, Meyers P, Huvos AG, et al. Improved outcomes in patients with osteogenic sarcoma of the head and neck. Cancer 2002;95(7):1495–503.
24. Fernandes R, Nikitakis NG, Pazoki A, et al. Osteogenic sarcoma of the jaw: a 10-year experience. J Oral Maxillofac Surg 2007;65(7):1286–91.
25. Huh WW, Holsinger FC, Levy A, et al. Osteosarcoma of the jaw in children and young adults. Head Neck 2012;34(7):981–4.
26. Batsakis JG, Mackay B, el-Naggar AK. Ewing's sarcoma and peripheral primitive neuroectodermal tumor: an interim report. Ann Otol Rhinol Laryngol 1996;105(10):838–43.
27. Jürgens H, Bier V, Harms D, et al. Malignant peripheral neuroectodermal tumors. A retrospective analysis of 42 patients. Cancer 1988;61(2):349–57.
28. Nikitakis NG, Salama AR, O'Malley BW, et al. Malignant peripheral primitive neuroectodermal tumor-peripheral neuroepithelioma of the head and neck: a clinicopathologic study of five cases and review of the literature. Head Neck 2003;25(6):488–98.

29. Jones JE, McGill T. Peripheral primitive neuroectodermal tumors of the head and neck. Arch Otolaryngol Head Neck Surg 1995;121(12):1392–5.

30. Alyahya GA, Heegaard S, Fledelius HC, et al. Primitive neuroectodermal tumor of the orbit in a 5-year-old girl with microphthalmia. Graefes Arch Clin Exp Ophthalmol 2000;238(9):801–6.

31. Whang-Peng J, Triche TJ, Knutsen T, et al. Chromosome translocation in peripheral neuroepithelioma. N Engl J Med 1984;311(9):584–5.

32. Vaccani JP, Forte V, de Jong AL, et al. Ewing's sarcoma of the head and neck in children. Int J Pediatr Otorhinolaryngol 1999;48(3):209–16.

33. Gradoni P, Giordano D, Oretti G, et al. Clinical outcomes of rhabdomyosarcoma and Ewing's sarcoma of the head and neck in children. Auris Nasus Larynx 2011;38(4):480–6.

34. Schuck A, Ahrens S, Paulussen M, et al. Local therapy in localized Ewing tumors: results of 1058 patients treated in the CESS 81, CESS 86, and EICESS 92 trials. Int J Radiat Oncol Biol Phys 2003;55(1):168–77.

35. Kruse-Lösler B, Gaertner C, Bürger H, et al. Melanotic neuroectodermal tumor of infancy: systematic review of the literature and presentation of a case. Oral Surg Oral Med Oral Pathol Oral Radiol Endod 2006;102(2):204–16.

36. Mosby EL, Lowe MW, Cobb CM, et al. Melanotic neuroectodermal tumor of infancy: review of the literature and report of a case. J Oral Maxillofac Surg 1992;50(8):886–94.

37. Judd PL, Harrop K, Becker J. Melanotic neuroectodermal tumor of infancy. Oral Surg Oral Med Oral Pathol 1990;69(6):723–6.

38. Rickert CH, Probst-Cousin S, Blasius S, et al. Melanotic progonoma of the brain: a case report and review. Childs Nerv Syst 1998;14(8):389–93.

39. De Chiara A, Van Tornout JM, Hachitanda Y, et al. Melanotic neuroectodermal tumor of infancy. A case report of paratesticular primary with lymph node involvement. Am J Pediatr Hematol Oncol 1992;14(4):356–60.

40. Demellawy DE, Young JL, Nanassy J, et al. Langerhans cell histiocytosis: a comprehensive review. Pathology 2015;47(4):294–301.

41. Lau L, Krafchik B, Trebo MM, et al. Cutaneous Langerhans cell histiocytosis in children under one year. Pediatr Blood Cancer 2006;46(1):66–71.

42. Bansal M, Srivastava VK, Bansal R, et al. Severe periodontal disease manifested in chronic disseminated type of Langerhans cell histiocytosis in a 3-year old child. Int J Clin Pediatr Dent 2014;7(3):217–9.

43. Lahey ME. Histiocytosis X: comparison of three treatment regimens. J Pediatr 1975;87(2):179–83.

44. da Costa CE, Annels NE, Faaij CM, et al. Presence of osteoclast-like multinucleated giant cells in the bone and nonostotic lesions of Langerhans cell histiocytosis. J Exp Med 2005;201(5):687–93.

45. Bouzourene H, Hutter P, Losi L, et al. Selection of patients with germline MLH1 mutated Lynch syndrome by determination of MLH1 methylation and BRAF mutation. Fam Cancer 2010;9(2):167–72.

46. Sozzi D, Morganti V, Valente GM, et al. Ameloblastic carcinoma in a young patient. Oral Surg Oral Med Oral Pathol Oral Radiol 2014;117(5):e396–402.

47. Yazici N, Karagöz B, Varan A, et al. Maxillary ameloblastic carcinoma in a child. Pediatr Blood Cancer 2008;50(1):175–6.

48. Van Dam SD, Unni KK, Keller EE. Metastasizing (malignant) ameloblastoma: review of a unique histopathologic entity and report of Mayo Clinic experience. J Oral Maxillofac Surg 2010;68(12):2962–74.

49. Berger AJ, Son J, Desai NK. Malignant ameloblastoma: concurrent presentation of primary and distant disease and review of the literature. J Oral Maxillofac Surg 2012;70(10):2316–26.

Pediatric Odontogenic Cysts of the Jaws

Kevin Arce, DMD, MD, MCR*, Christopher S. Streff, DDS, MD, Kyle S. Ettinger, DDS, MD

KEYWORDS

- Odontogenic cysts • Maxillofacial surgery • Pediatrics • Diagnosis • Treatment

KEY POINTS

- Cysts have characteristically 3 main features: the presence of an epithelial lining, a centrally located lumen, and a surrounding connective tissue wall.
- Jaw cysts are broadly categorized as either odontogenic or nonodontogenic based on the type of tissue from which the epithelial lining derives from.
- Odontogenic cysts are further subclassified as either inflammatory or developmental depending on the cause.
- Pediatric odontogenic cysts are predominantly periapical (radicular) cysts, buccal bifurcation cysts, eruption cysts, and dentigerous cysts.
- The common pediatric odontogenic cysts are amenable to simple treatment and have an overall excellent prognosis with a low recurrence rate.

INTRODUCTION

All pathologic cysts are characteristically unified by 3 salient features: the presence of an epithelial lining, a centrally located lumen, and a surrounding connective tissue wall. A multitude of cystic lesions are well known to occur within the jaws, and it is of critical importance for oral and maxillofacial surgeons to have an understanding of the clinicopathologic presentation, management, and natural history of each of these entities. Cysts involving the jaws are broadly categorized as either odontogenic or nonodontogenic based on the type of tissue from which the epithelial lining derives (**Box 1**). Odontogenic cysts are further subclassified as either inflammatory or developmental depending on their underlying cause (see **Box 1**). Historically, the classification of odontogenic cysts has been a treatise on controversy and debate.[1–4] Some entities previously described

as odontogenic cysts have more recently been reclassified into other pathologic categories (ie, odontogenic keratocyst [OKC] and calcifying odontogenic cyst [COC]).[5] Other historical entities have been completely dispelled through more refined histologic characterization (ie, the primordial cyst).[5] Of the currently accepted subtypes of odontogenic cysts, only a limited number are well known to occur in pediatric populations (**Box 2**). This article provides an in-depth accounting of the epidemiology, clinical/radiographic features, histopathology, treatment, and prognosis for each of these odontogenic cysts. Other odontogenic cysts that rarely present in pediatric populations are addressed but are not covered in significant detail. Similarly, odontogenic cysts that have controversially been redesignated as odontogenic neoplasms are covered only in limited detail, as they are addressed in other articles in this issue.

Disclosure Statement: The authors have nothing to disclose.

Division of Oral and Maxillofacial Surgery, Department of Surgery, Mayo College of Medicine, Mayo Clinic, 200 First Street Southwest, Ro_ma_12_12econ, Rochester, MN 55901, USA

* Corresponding author.

E-mail address: arce.kevin@mayo.edu

Oral Maxillofacial Surg Clin N Am 28 (2016) 21–30

http://dx.doi.org/10.1016/j.coms.2015.07.003

Box 1
Classification of cysts involving the jaws

Odontogenic
- Inflammatory
  - Periapical (radicular) cyst[a]
  - Buccal bifurcation cyst
- Developmental
  - Dentigerous cyst
  - Eruption cyst
  - Glandular odontogenic cyst
  - Lateral periodontal cyst
  - Gingival cyst of the adult
  - Calcifying odontogenic cyst[b]
  - Odontogenic keratocyst[b]

Nonodontogenic
- Nasopalatine duct cyst
- Median palatine cyst
- Nasolabial cyst
- Gingival cyst of the newborn
- Palatal cysts of the newborn
  - Epstein pearls
  - Bohn nodules

[a]Includes residual periapical (radicular) cysts and lateral radicular cysts.
[b]Both are classified as odontogenic tumors according to the most recent World Health Organization Classification of Head and Neck Tumors.[5]

PERIAPICAL (RADICULAR) CYST

Periapical or radicular cysts are inflammatory cysts that form at the apices of endodontically compromised teeth. True radicular cysts are believed to originate from an inflammatory-

Box 2
Pediatric odontogenic cysts

Inflammatory
- Periapical (radicular) cysts[a]
- Buccal bifurcation cyst

Developmental
- Dentigerous cyst
- Eruption cyst

[a]Includes residual periapical (radicular) cysts and lateral radicular cysts.

mediated proliferation of normally quiescent epithelial nests (epithelial rests of Malassez) that are present in the apical periodontal ligament spaces.[6–8] When considering patients of all age groups, radicular cysts are the most common subtype of cyst affecting the jaws and they comprise approximately 52% to 68% of cysts presenting within this anatomic region.[7] The incidence of radicular cysts is reported to be the highest in the third decade of life[7]; however, epidemiologic studies on radicular cysts specifically within pediatric populations are lacking. Although radicular cysts are more commonly associated with endodontically compromised permanent teeth, they have also been described in a limited number of cases involving deciduous teeth.[8,9] Based on the limited number of cases reported in the literature, radicular cysts associated with primary teeth are believed to represent less than 1% of all radicular cysts.[8] However, the actual prevalence is likely higher than the literature suggests given the propensity for clinicians to neglect radiolucencies involving primary teeth and the eventual resolution of the lesion once the primary tooth is either exfoliated or extracted.[8,9]

Clinically, radicular cysts involving permanent teeth can occur in any tooth-bearing area of the jaws; however, they are reported to occur more frequently in the maxilla with a predilection for the anterior maxillary dentition.[7] In the mandible, radicular cysts are reported to occur most frequently in the premolar region.[7] Radicular cysts involving deciduous teeth are known to most commonly occur in association with the primary mandibular molars.[8,9] Patients typically endorse symptoms consistent with the natural history of a pulpitis, as radicular cysts are considered to be the direct sequelae to apical granulomas that form in the wake of endodontic infection.[7] However, not all periapical granulomas progress to radicular cysts. Because radicular cysts represent chronic inflammatory lesions, they are typically asymptomatic by the time they become well developed. Teeth associated with radicular cysts are classically nonresponsive to vitality testing, and depending on the size of the cyst tooth mobility can occasionally be noted. Radiographically, radicular cysts are indistinguishable from periapical granulomas, and unfortunately, there are no discrete imaging characteristics to distinguish between these 2 separate pathologic entities. Lateral radicular cysts and residual periapical cysts are both terms used to describe different radiographic presentations of radicular cysts. The former is located at the lateral aspect of the root of a nonvital tooth, and the latter is found in the area of a previous extraction site.

Histologically, radicular cysts arising from permanent teeth or deciduous teeth are virtually indistinguishable.[9] The characteristic findings in radicular cysts are the presence of a dense fibrous connective tissue wall, a nonkeratinized stratified squamous epithelial lining, and a histologically evident lumen.[7,9] Heavy inflammatory cell infiltrates are often seen throughout both the connective tissue wall and the lining epithelium.[9] Fluid or cellular debris can be seen occupying the lumen of the integrity of the cyst is not disrupted at the time of removal. Two histologic variants of radicular cysts have been reported, the periapical pocket cyst and the periapical true cyst.[7] The periapical pocket cyst is characterized by an epithelium-lined cavity that remains open to the root apex of the affected tooth, whereas the epithelium of a true cyst remains adjacent to and completely separated from the tooth apex.[7]

Treatment of radicular cysts proceeds in a fashion identical to the management of all periapical radiolucencies. Vitality testing should always be performed to confirm the presence of a necrotic pulp. Treatment can then proceed with either endodontic therapy or extraction of the tooth if indicated. Any periapical lesion that remains persistent after nonsurgical root canal therapy should always be interrogated either by endodontic retreatment if the initial therapy was believed to be insufficient or by surgical intervention in the form of apical surgery or extraction of the tooth. Although some investigators suggest that periapical pocket cysts can be effectively managed through nonsurgical endodontic therapy alone (given the confluence of the cyst epithelium with the apex of the tooth), most studies suggesting this are based purely on physiologic extrapolation rather than rigorous scientific method.[6,7] Ultimately, true radicular cysts are not responsive to root canal therapy given their isolation from the root canal system, and surgical intervention in the form of curettement is invariably required for resolution (**Fig. 1**).[6,7]

Prognosis for radicular cysts is excellent presuming adequate surgical management. With the cause of radicular cysts being of an inflammatory nature, the rates of recurrence are essentially zero if the entirety of the cyst is

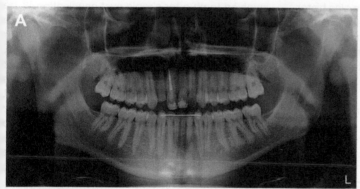

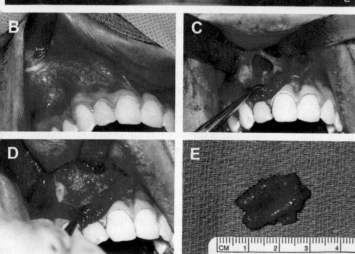

Fig. 1. Large radicular cyst presenting in a 17-year-old boy. (*A*) Panoramic radiograph demonstrating persistent corticated periapical radiolucency after endodontic treatment of tooth No. 8. (*B–D*) Surgical enucleation of cyst with allogeneic bone grafting of defect. (*E*) Removed specimen.

removed and the source of the inflammation is appropriately treated.

BUCCAL BIFURCATION CYST

Buccal bifurcation cysts represent a rare form of inflammatory odontogenic cyst that has historically been known by several pseudonyms, including mandibular infected buccal cyst in the molar area, circumferential dentigerous cyst, inflammatory collateral dental cyst, inflammatory paradental cyst, and juvenile paradental cyst.[10,11] To date approximately 63 cases of buccal bifurcation cysts have been reported within the literature through various case reports and cases series.[10–15] All described buccal bifurcation cysts have been reported to occur in association with either the mandibular first or mandibular second permanent molars.[11,16] The typical age of onset is between 4 and 14 years, as this time frame corresponds to the eruption of each of these respective teeth.[11,16] The true cause for the inflammatory response leading to cyst formation remains unclear. Some have postulated that cusp perforation through the oral mucosa during tooth eruption may represent a potential mechanism for formation.[11,17] Alternative explanations have also historically included the presence of enamel projections extending from the cementoenamel junction to the furcation area of the tooth. However, this theory remains questionable as most reported cases do not present with this feature.[17]

Clinically, buccal bifurcation cysts present with a classic array of findings: involvement of partially erupted vital first or second molar, buccal soft-tissue swelling, delayed or altered eruption of the involved tooth, and an increase in periodontal pocket depth in the affected area.[10,16] Several radiographic findings are also classically present: a radiolucent lesion located on the buccal aspect of the affected tooth, tilting of the involved molar with the root apices pointing toward the mandibular lingual cortex, an intact periodontal ligament space and lamina dura, extension of the radiolucent lesion to the inferior border of the mandible without alteration in the osseous anatomy of the inferior cortex, and a periosteal reaction on the buccal surface of the mandible (varying from a single layer to an onion-skin appearance).[10,16]

Histologically, buccal bifurcation cysts demonstrate an epithelial lining composed of nonkeratinized stratified squamous epithelium with focal areas of hyperplasia.[10,16,17] There is often a dense inflammatory infiltrate involving both the connective tissue wall and the lining epithelium of the cyst,[10,16,17] which is analogous to the histologic findings seen in other types of inflammatory

odontogenic cysts (ie, radicular cysts, residual periapical cysts, lateral radicular cysts).

The treatment of buccal bifurcation cysts has continued to evolve with time. Historically, buccal bifurcation cysts were managed with extraction of the involved tooth and enucleation of the cyst.[10,17] Subsequent studies have demonstrated that extraction of the tooth is unnecessary and simple cyst enucleation is sufficient treatment.[17] Less invasive nonsurgical strategies involving periodontal probing and daily periodontal pocket irrigation have been more recently suggested as an alternative to enucleation.[11] These nonsurgical regimens have been tried only in a limited number of cases, and therefore cyst enucleation without tooth extraction remains the current treatment modality of choice.[10,11]

Prognosis for buccal bifurcation cysts after enucleation is excellent. In the largest prospective series on outcomes for buccal bifurcation cyst, no recurrences were noted after cyst enucleation and maintenance of the involved teeth.[16] This same study also demonstrated normalization of aberrant eruption patterns, adequate radiographic fill of osseous defects, normalization of periodontal probing depths, and maintained vitality of all involved teeth after simple cyst enucleation.[16]

DENTIGEROUS CYST

Dentigerous cysts arise from the follicle of an impacted or a developing tooth. These cysts are the second most common odontogenic cyst, with a reported male predilection and an estimated frequency of 1.44 in every 100 impacted teeth.[18–20] They occur over a wide age range, with the highest incidence in the second to fourth decade of life. Dentigerous cysts are commonly associated with impacted mandibular third molars, followed by the maxillary permanent canines, mandibular second premolars, and maxillary third molars.[19]

The dentigerous cyst develops by accumulation of fluid between the reduced enamel epithelium and the crown or between the layers of the enamel epithelium.[18] The exact histogenesis of dentigerous cysts remains unclear, with most investigators favoring a developmental origin. An inflammatory type has also been described, with clinical presentation and demographics that differ from those of its counterpart.[1,19,21] The developmental dentigerous cyst occurs mainly in the permanent dentition and in association with an impacted mandibular third molar. Patients are typically in their second to third decade of life and are asymptomatic, unless the cyst becomes secondarily infected. The inflammatory type occurs in the developing permanent teeth as a result of inflammation from a nonvital deciduous tooth that spreads to involve the underlying tooth follicle and stimulates the separation and fluid accumulation between the reduced enamel epithelium and the crown. These cysts are diagnosed earlier, in the first and early part of the second decade, and patients present with swelling and pain. The mandibular premolars are commonly involved seemingly because of the higher caries susceptibility of the deciduous molar and proximity of its roots to the follicle of the succedaneous teeth.[22]

Dentigerous cysts are characteristically asymptomatic and noted during routine radiographic evaluation. The presence of a well-circumscribed, unilocular radiolucency around the crown of an impacted or developing tooth is considered a classic finding in the formulation of a differential diagnosis that includes this entity. In a developing tooth, the size of the radiolucent lesion must be larger than that of the dental follicle, which is considered normal in size when less than 4 mm.[18] Dentigerous cysts can become large and lead to displacement of the associated impacted tooth, root resorption of the adjacent dentition, and bone resorption (**Fig. 2**).

Histologically, they are lined by a thin, nonkeratinizing, stratified squamous epithelium. The lining can resemble the reduced enamel epithelium, and mucous cells may be present. Focal epithelial hyperplasia of varying thickness may occur because of secondary inflammation and may make dentigerous cysts histologically indistinguishable from a radicular cyst.[19] The following criteria have been recommended for establishing the diagnosis of a dentigerous cyst: (1) presence of pericoronal radiolucency larger than 4 mm in greatest dimension, (2) histologic finding of a nonkeratinized, stratified squamous epithelium, and (3) the presence of a cystic space between the enamel and the overlying tissue at the time of the surgical intervention.[18]

Treatment of dentigerous cysts is complete surgical enucleation and extraction of the associated impacted tooth. When a developing permanent tooth is present, decompression or marsupialization may be performed after obtaining histopathologic confirmation to aid in the eruption of the tooth. This treatment helps maintain the developing dentition and minimizes injury to adjacent structures.[23–26] When marsupialization or decompression is used for large lesions, there is

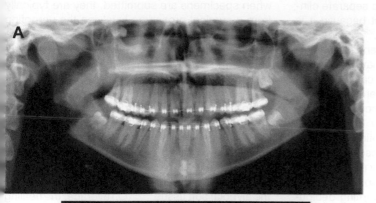

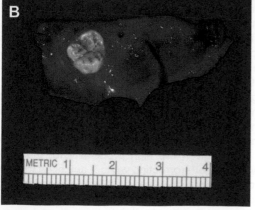

Fig. 2. Dentigerous cyst presenting in a 17-year-old girl. (*A*) Panoramic radiograph depicting severely displaced impacted tooth No. 1 secondary to a cystic lesion involving the right maxillary sinus. (*B*) Path specimen after tooth extraction and concomitant cyst enucleation.

variability in treatment time and the possibility of requiring a secondary procedure to remove any remaining tissue or providing orthodontic traction for eruption of an impacted tooth.[23] The identified factors that influence the eruption of an impacted tooth associated with a dentigerous cyst without orthodontic traction are (1) the age of a patient (<10 years), (2) depth of impaction in relationship to the adjacent cementoenamel junction and cusp tip (<5.1 mm), (3) angulation less than 25%, and (4) space to tooth ratio greater than 1:1.[27] The successful eruption of an impacted tooth associated with a dentigerous cyst can be predicted within the first 3 months after marsupialization, and orthodontic traction could be considered at that point if progress is not observed.[28]

The prognosis for dentigerous cysts is excellent given that recurrence is extremely rare after definitive treatment. Enucleation alone is curative, and the use of adjuvant treatment modalities is not required.

ERUPTION CYST

Eruption cysts represent a variant of dentigerous cyst that develops in the soft tissue just before a tooth erupts into the oral cavity. This cyst originates from the separation of the dental follicle from the crown of the tooth as it erupts through the soft tissue. It is recognized as a separate clinical entity from a dentigerous cyst because it is confined to the alveolar soft tissue.[29,30] The exact cause of eruption cysts has not been clearly identified within the literature. Studies have suggested that stimulation of soft tissue, early caries, trauma, infection, and deficient space for eruption are all possible causes.[29,31] The prevalence of eruption cysts reported in the literature is low. Potential reasons for this are that most eruption cysts are asymptomatic and frequently resolve without treatment; thus, most patients likely never present to a health care provider.[29] An eruption cyst can develop in association with any erupting deciduous or permanent tooth. These cysts are most frequently reported to occur in the permanent dentition between ages 6 and 9 years, as this age range coincides with the eruption of the permanent incisors and first molars.[31,32] Heterogeneity exists in reports of the most common location for eruption cysts to occur. Some studies suggest that the highest frequency is in the permanent incisor and first molar region, whereas others report the highest incidence in the permanent canine and premolar region.[29–32]

Clinically, eruption cysts present as a well-circumscribed, fluctuant lesion in the alveolar soft tissue overlying an erupting tooth. The color of this cystic lesion can range from translucent to bluish-purple or even dark bluish-black hue.[31] The darker clinical appearance represents blood within the cystic cavity and is often referred to as an eruption hematoma. The presenting size of the eruption cyst depends on the size of the underlying tooth, with permanent teeth presenting with larger cyst formation.[29,32] Eruption cysts typically present as isolated unilateral occurrences, but multiple eruption cysts and bilateral presentations have also been reported.[33] Most of these lesions are asymptomatic but can become symptomatic because of trauma or a secondary infection.[29] Given that the cyst itself is isolated to the soft tissue, there are few characteristic radiographic findings. An erupting tooth should always be radiographically evident underlying the involved area, and there should be no evidence of an intraosseous component to the cyst. In contrast, a dentigerous cyst is radiographically evident surrounding the crown of a nonerupting tooth and can have osseous involvement.[29,34]

Histologically, the eruption cyst is derived from the reduced enamel epithelium. The lining of the cyst is composed of a nonkeratinized stratified squamous epithelium. Because surgical intervention is seldom required for the management of these cysts, histopathologic specimens are not frequently submitted for review. Nevertheless, when specimens are submitted, they are typically from a surgical procedure involving the unroofing of the cystic cavity to facilitate eruption of the underlying tooth. Accordingly, these specimens typically demonstrate normal-appearing oral mucosa superficially, a variable thickness of intervening lamina propria, and the cystic cavity lined with of a thin layer of nonkeratinized squamous epithelium at the deepest margin of the specimen.

The vast majority of eruption cysts do not require surgical intervention. They remain asymptomatic and naturally automarsupialize as the underlying tooth erupts into the cystic space and then through the alveolar soft tissue.[29,31] On average, the healing of an asymptomatic eruption cyst is approximately 5 weeks.[31] Less commonly, eruption cysts can continue to enlarge, leading to pain and swelling in the area. If an eruption cyst becomes secondarily infected, then surgical management with an incision over the cyst in the gingival crest would be indicated. This treatment allows the cyst to marsupialize into the oral cavity and for the tooth to continue to erupt into proper position.[29,30]

The prognosis for eruption cysts is excellent given the high propensity for these cysts to be self-correcting without any need for surgical intervention. Given this, the likelihood for recurrence is essentially nil on appropriate eruption of the offending tooth into the oral cavity.

ODONTOGENIC CYSTS UNCOMMON IN PEDIATRIC POPULATIONS
Glandular Odontogenic Cyst

A glandular odontogenic cyst (GOC) is a rare, locally aggressive cyst with a known high propensity for recurrence. GOC comprises less than 1% of all odontogenic cysts, with only 114 cases reported in the literature and only 9 reported cases involving pediatric patients.[35–37] GOCs typically present in the fifth to sixth decades of life with a mean age of onset of 45 years.[35] Approximately 75% of these GOCs occur in the mandible with a specific predilection for the anterior mandible. Cysts involving the maxilla most commonly involve the anterior region.[35] The clinical presentation depends on the size and location of the cyst; however, an asymptomatic swelling represents the most common initial finding. Large cysts are known to present with localized pain or paresthesia.[35,38] Radiographically, these GOCs appear as unilocular or multilocular radiolucencies with well-defined sclerotic borders. Tooth resorption and/or tooth displacement can be seen. Histologically, GOC can present with a multitude of different findings, which can make accurate diagnosis a challenge.[39] Typically, the epithelial lining is composed of nonkeratinized stratified squamous epithelium with variable thickness and areas of focal luminal proliferation including epithelial whorls and spheres.[39] Cuboidal eosinophilic cells are often seen superficially in the epithelial lining.[39] Mucous cells can be seen superficially in the epithelial lining, and intraepithelial ductlike structures can also be appreciated. These latter findings can lead to an inappropriate diagnosis of mucoepidermoid carcinoma if reviewed by less experienced pathologists; however, immunohistochemical studies are valuable in differentiating between these 2 entities.[35,39] Treatment of GOCs varies depending on the clinical presentation of the lesion. Small unilocular lesions are amenable to enucleation and curettage. However, larger multilocular lesions typically require more aggressive treatment strategies such as enucleation with peripheral ostectomy, marginal resection, or even segmental resection if the cysts have grown to large proportions. Recurrence rates for GOC have been reported to be as high as 29% to 50% with enucleation and curettage alone; however, this rate decreases significantly when more aggressive treatment strategies are used.[40,41]

Lateral Periodontal Cyst

Lateral periodontal cysts (LPCs) are rare noninflammatory odontogenetic cysts that comprise approximately 1% of all odontogenic cysts.[37,42] LPCs are thought to derive from vestigial cell rests originating from the dental lamina.[43] This cyst is extremely rare in pediatric populations, with only a few documented pediatric cases within the literature.[44,45] LPCs predominantly affect adults, with the average age of onset in the fifth to sixth decades of life.[46] The most commonly involved area of the oral cavity is in the mandibular premolar region followed by the anterior maxilla. LPCs are generally asymptomatic and are often incidentally identified during routine dental care.[47,48] Radiographically, these lesions present as a well-circumscribed radiolucency with a sclerotic border adjacent to the root of a vital tooth. The periodontal ligament space is not enlarged, and it is uncommon for these cysts to grow larger than 1 cm in diameter.[49] Histologically, LPCs are lined with nonkeratinized squamous epithelium and epithelial plaques are often visible throughout the specimen.[47,50] LPCs do not demonstrate any inflammatory infiltrate in the lining epithelium or in the cyst wall. Diagnosis of the lesion can be confirmed only through biopsy and histopathologic review as no distinct clinical or radiographic findings can differentiate LPCs from other cystic lesions. The recommended treatment involves surgical enucleation with preservation of the adjacent tooth. Recurrence rates for LPCs after simple enucleation are reported to be exceedingly low.[49]

Gingival Cyst of the Adult

Gingival cyst of the adult (GCOA) represents the soft-tissue counterpart of the LPC. GCOA is an extremely rare pathologic entity representing less than 0.5% of all odontogenic cysts.[51] As the name suggests, these cysts predominantly present in adult populations and are most commonly reported to occur during the fourth to fifth decades of life.[51] Review of the literature revealed an isolated case report of a GCOA occurring in a 16-year-old boy[51]; however, given the overwhelming rarity of this lesion in pediatric populations, it is not discussed in any further detail.

ODONTOGENIC CYSTS CLASSIFIED AS ODONTOGENIC NEOPLASMS
Odontogenic Keratocyst

The classification of odontogenic keratocysts (OKCs) has historically been an area of fervent debate among oral and maxillofacial surgeons, and the discourse remains ongoing.[4] Although the World Health Organization (WHO) classifies the OKC as the keratocystic odontogenic tumor (KCOT), this terminology has not yet been universally adopted by the scientific community.[4,5] The basis for the reclassification of OKC as KCOT stems from the aggressive clinical behavior of the lesion, specific histologic features suggestive of neoplastic tendencies (eg, epithelial budding into connective tissue, mitotic figures in suprabasal layers of epithelial lining), and the genetic association with tumor suppressor gene PTCH and the oncogene SMO (present in both sporadic KCOTs and in KCOTs associated with nevoid basal cell carcinoma syndrome).[52] The specific details regarding the controversy of OKC reclassification as KCOT are beyond the scope of this article, and the description of OKC as a pathologic entity is covered in further detail in other articles in this issue.

Calcifying Odontogenic Cyst

The COC, not unlike the OKC, represents yet another odontogenic cyst that has been controversially reclassified as an odontogenic neoplasm under the current WHO guidelines.[5] COC was first described by Gorlin and colleagues[53] in 1962, and since then there have been several hundred documented reports within the literature.[54] No definitive consensus exists regarding the classification of COCs as a cyst or a neoplasm, owing in part to its widely variable clinicopathologic presentation and biological behavior.[55] Under the most recent WHO guidelines COC has been reclassified as the calcifying cystic odontogenic tumor and represents a single constituent of the larger spectrum of ghost cell odontogenic tumors, which also includes dentinogenic ghost cell tumor and ghost cell odontogenic carcinoma.[5,54] Overall, COCs represent uncommon lesions, comprising approximately 5% to 7% of all odontogenic tumors.[56] COCs most commonly arise in individuals during the second and third decades of life; however, they are also known to occur in pediatric populations, particularly in association with odontomas.[54,57]

Clinically, COCs most commonly present as an asymptomatic swelling, although pain and displacement of teeth have also been reported.[56] They are known to occur in equal frequency in the maxilla and mandible, with a specific predilection for anterior canine to incisor regions.[56] Radiographically, COCs present as mixed lesions with a well-defined radiolucent component and scattered areas of radiopaque foci.[56] Up to one-third of cases occur in association with impacted teeth or odontomas.[54,56] Extraosseous COCs can also occur and typically resemble other types of gingival swellings (ie, gingival fibromas, peripheral giant cell granulomas).[54]

Histologically, COCs are composed of a cystic cavity that is lined by stratified odontogenic epithelium of variable thickness.[54,57] The epithelial lining is often composed of a well-defined columnar basal cell layer resembling ameloblasts; however, stellate reticulum-like cells, ghost cells and undifferentiated epithelium resembling reduced enamel epithelium can also be present in varying quantities.[54,57] The lesion is often surrounded by a thick connective tissue capsule and an inflammatory foreign body reaction is typically present.[56] In addition to the cystic components, COCs can also demonstrate variable amounts of solid luminal and/or mural proliferations that have an ameloblastomatous appearance.[56]

Treatment of COCs involves conservative surgery with enucleation and curettage.[54,56,57] Prognosis for central COC after simple enucleation and curettage is excellent, with extremely low recurrence rates reported across numerous series.[54,56,57] The prognosis for extraosseous COCs is also excellent with minimal likelihood of recurrence following simple surgical excision.[54]

SUMMARY

Odontogenic cysts represent a common form of pathology that virtually every oral and maxillofacial surgeon should possess a thorough understanding of in terms of natural history, clinicopathologic findings, and appropriate management strategies. Odontogenic cysts arising in pediatric populations, although less numerous than those presenting in adults, are nevertheless important pathologic entities that oral and maxillofacial surgeons should be adequately equipped to address. Categorizing pediatric odontogenic cysts into either inflammatory or developmental causesprovides a convenient way of conceptualizing these various entities and can facilitate the appropriate diagnosis and subsequent management.

REFERENCES

1. Main DM. Epithelial jaw cysts: 10 years of the WHO classification. J Oral Pathol 1985;14(1):1–7.
2. Regezi JA, Courtney RM, Batsakis JG. The pathology of head and neck tumors: cysts of the jaws, part 12. Head Neck Surg 1981;4(1):48–57.
3. Daley TE, Wysocki GP. New developments in selected cysts of the jaws. J Can Dent Assoc 1997;63(7):526–7, 530–2.
4. Bhargava D, Deshpande A, Pogrel MA. Keratocystic odontogenic tumour (KCOT)–a cyst to a tumour. Oral Maxillofac Surg 2012;16(2):163–70.
5. Barnes L. Universitäts-Spital Zurich. Department Pathologie, International Academy of Pathology, World Health Organization, International Agency

for Research on Cancer. Pathology and genetics of head and neck tumours. Lyon (France): IARC Press; 2007.

6. Lin LM, Huang GT, Rosenberg PA. Proliferation of epithelial cell rests, formation of apical cysts, and regression of apical cysts after periapical wound healing. J Endod 2007;33(8):908–16.

7. Nair PN. New perspectives on radicular cysts: do they heal? Int Endod J 1998;31(3):155–60.

8. Shetty S, Angadi PV, Rekha K. Radicular cyst in deciduous maxillary molars: a rarity. Head Neck Pathol 2010;4(1):27–30.

9. Mass E, Kaplan I, Hirshberg A. A clinical and histopathological study of radicular cysts associated with primary molars. J Oral Pathol Med 1995; 24(10):458–61.

10. Levarek RE, Wiltz MJ, Kelsch RD, et al. Surgical management of the buccal bifurcation cyst: bone grafting as a treatment adjunct to enucleation and curettage. J Oral Maxillofac Surg 2014;72(10): 1966–73.

11. Ramos LM, Vargas PA, Coletta RD, et al. Bilateral buccal bifurcation cyst: case report and literature review. Head Neck Pathol 2012;6(4):455–9.

12. Boffano P, Gallesio C, Roccia F, et al. Bilateral buccal bifurcation cyst. J Craniofac Surg 2012; 23(6):e643–5.

13. Borgonovo AE, Reo P, Grossi GB, et al. Paradental cyst of the first molar: report of a rare case with bilateral presentation and review of the literature. J Indian Soc Pedod Prev Dent 2012;30(4):343–8.

14. Borgonovo AE, Rigaldo F, Censi R, et al. Large buccal bifurcation cyst in a child: a case report and literature review. Eur J Paediatr Dent 2014; 15(2 Suppl):237–40.

15. Friedrich RE, Scheuer HA, Zustin J. Inflammatory paradental cyst of the first molar (buccal bifurcation cyst) in a 6-year-old boy: case report with respect to immunohistochemical findings. In Vivo 2014;28(3): 333–9.

16. Pompura JR, Sandor GK, Stoneman DW. The buccal bifurcation cyst: a prospective study of treatment outcomes in 44 sites. Oral Surg Oral Med Oral Pathol Oral Radiol Endod 1997;83(2):215–21.

17. Corona-Rodriguez J, Torres-Labardini R, Velasco-Tizcareno M, et al. Bilateral buccal bifurcation cyst: case report and literature review. J Oral Maxillofac Surg 2011;69(6):1694–6.

18. Daley TD, Wysocki GP. The small dentigerous cyst: a diagnostic dilemma. Oral Surg Oral Med Oral Pathol Oral Radiol Endod 1995;79(1):77–81.

19. Benn A, Altini M. Dentigerous cysts of inflammatory origin: a clinicopathologic study. Oral Surg Oral Med Oral Pathol Oral Radiol Endod 1996;81(2):203–9.

20. Mourshed F. A roentgenographic study of dentigerous cysts: I. incidence in a population sample. Oral Surg Oral Med Oral Pathol 1964;18(1):47–53.

21. Bloch-Jorgensen K. Follicular cysts. Dental Cosmos 1928;70:708–11.

22. Shibata Y, Asaumi J, Yanagi Y, et al. Radiographic examination of dentigerous cysts in the transitional dentition. Dentomaxillofac Radiol 2004;33(1):17–20.

23. Allon DM, Allon I, Anavi Y, et al. Decompression as a treatment of odontogenic cystic lesions in children. J Oral Maxillofac Surg 2015;73(4):649–54.

24. Hu Y-H, Chang Y-L, Tsai A. Conservative treatment of dentigerous cyst associated with primary teeth. Oral Surg Oral Med Oral Pathol Oral Radiol Endod 2011; 112(6):e5–7.

25. Huseyin K, Esin A, Aycan K. Outcome of dentigerous cysts treated with marsupialization. J Clin Pediatr Dent 2009;34(2):165–8.

26. Wiemer SJ, Pruitt CA, Rallis DJ, et al. Use of a modified removable partial denture as a marsupialization stent in a pediatric patient. J Oral Maxillofac Surg 2013;71(8):1382–6.

27. Fujii R, Kawakami M, Hyomoto M, et al. Panoramic findings for predicting eruption of mandibular premolars associated with dentigerous cyst after marsupialization. J Oral Maxillofac Surg 2008;66(2):272–6.

28. Yahara Y, Kubota Y, Yamashiro T, et al. Eruption prediction of mandibular premolars associated with dentigerous cysts. Oral Surg Oral Med Oral Pathol Oral Radiol Endod 2009;108(1):28–31.

29. Anderson R. Eruption cysts: a retrograde study. ASDC J Dent Child 1989;57(2):124–7.

30. Nagaveni NB, Umashankara KV, Radhika NB, et al. Eruption cyst: a literature review and four case reports. Indian J Dent Res 2011;22(1):148–51.

31. Aguilo L, Cibrian R, Bagan JV, et al. Eruption cysts: retrospective clinical study of 36 cases. ASDC J Dent Child 1998;65(2):102–6.

32. Bodner L, Goldstein J, Sarnat H. Eruption cysts: a clinical report of 24 new cases. J Clin Pediatr Dentistry 2005;28(2):183–6.

33. Ramon Boj J, Garcia-Godoy F. Multiple eruption cysts: report of case. ASDC J Dent Child 2000; 67(4):282–4, 232.

34. Dhawan P, Kochhar GK, Chachra S, et al. Eruption cysts: a series of two cases. Dental Res J 2012; 9(5):647.

35. Mascitti M, Santarelli A, Sabatucci A, et al. Glandular odontogenic cyst: review of literature and report of a new case with cytokeratin-19 expression. Open Dent J 2014;8:1–12.

36. Tambawala SS, Karjodkar FR, Yadav A, et al. Glandular odontogenic cyst: a case report. Imaging Sci Dent 2014;44(1):75–9.

37. Sharifian MJ, Khalili M. Odontogenic cysts: a retrospective study of 1227 cases in an Iranian population from 1987 to 2007. J Oral Sci 2011;53(3):361–7.

38. Shah M, Kale H, Ranginwala A, et al. Glandular odontogenic cyst: a rare entity. J Oral Maxillofac Pathol 2014;18(1):89–92.

39. Kaplan I, Anavi Y, Hirshberg A. Glandular odonto-genic cyst: a challenge in diagnosis and treatment. Oral Dis 2008;14(7):575–81.

40. Kaplan I, Gal G, Anavi Y, et al. Glandular odonto-genic cyst: treatment and recurrence. J Oral Maxillo-fac Surg 2005;63(4):435–41.

41. Fowler CB, Brannon RB, Kessler HP, et al. Glandular odontogenic cyst: analysis of 46 cases with special emphasis on microscopic criteria for diagnosis. Head Neck Pathol 2011;5(4):364–75.

42. Shear M. Developmental odontogenic cysts. An up-date. J Oral Pathol Med 1994;23(1):1–11.

43. Wysocki GP, Brannon RB, Gardner DG, et al. Histo-genesis of the lateral periodontal cyst and the gingival cyst of the adult. Oral Surg Oral Med Oral Pathol 1980;50(4):327–34.

44. Govil S, Gupta V, Misra N, et al. Bilateral lateral peri-odontal cyst. BMJ Case Rep 2013;2013. p. 1–3.

45. Yang Y, Xia X, Wang W, et al. Uncommon fusion of teeth and lateral periodontal cyst in a Chinese girl: a case report. Oral Surg Oral Med Oral Pathol Oral Radiol Endod 2011;112(4):e18–20.

46. Altini M, Shear M. The lateral periodontal cyst: an update. J Oral Pathol Med 1992;21(6):245–50.

47. de Carvalho LF, Lima CF, Cabral LA, et al. Lateral periodontal cyst: a case report and literature review. J Oral Maxillofac Res 2011;1(4):e5.

48. Cohen DA, Neville BW, Damm DD, et al. The lateral periodontal cyst. A report of 37 cases. J Periodontol 1984;55(4):230–4.

49. Rasmusson LG, Magnusson BC, Borrman H. The lateral periodontal cyst. A histopathological and radiographic study of 32 cases. Br J Oral Maxillofac Surg 1991;29(1):54–7.

50. Friedrich RE, Scheuer HA, Zustin J. Lateral peri-odontal cyst. In Vivo 2014;28(4):595–8.

51. Malali VV, Satisha TS, Jha AK, et al. Gingival cyst of adult: a rare case. J Indian Soc Periodontol 2012; 16(3):465–8.

52. Madras J, Lapointe H. Keratocystic odontogenic tumour: reclassification of the odontogenic kerato-cyst from cyst to tumour. J Can Dent Assoc 2008; 74(2). 165–165h.

53. Gorlin RJ, Pindborg JJ, Odont, et al. The calcifying odontogenic cyst–a possible analogue of the cuta-neous calcifying epithelioma of Malherbe. An anal-ysis of fifteen cases. Oral Surg Oral Med Oral Pathol 1962;15:1235–43.

54. Lee SK, Kim YS. Current concepts and occurrence of epithelial odontogenic tumors: II. Calcifying epithelial odontogenic tumor versus ghost cell odon-togenic tumors derived from calcifying odontogenic cyst. Korean J Pathol 2014;48(3):175–87.

55. Toida M. So-called calcifying odontogenic cyst: re-view and discussion on the terminology and classifi-cation. J Oral Pathol Med 1998;27(2):49–52.

56. Fregnani ER, Pires FR, Quezada RD, et al. Calcifying odontogenic cyst: clinicopathological features and immunohistochemical profile of 10 cases. J Oral Pathol Med 2003;32(3):163–70.

57. Li TJ, Yu SF. Clinicopathologic spectrum of the so-called calcifying odontogenic cysts: a study of 21 intraosseous cases with reconsideration of the termi-nology and classification. Am J Surg Pathol 2003; 27(3):372–84.

Nonodontogenic Cysts of the Jaws and Treatment in the Pediatric Population

Richard Scott Jones, DDS[a], Jasjit Dillon, MBBS, DDS, FDSRCS[b],*

KEYWORDS

- Pediatric • Nonodontogenic • Cysts • Jaws

KEY POINTS

- Nonodontogenic cysts within the jaws are not a common presentation, especially in the pediatric population.
- It is well documented that cysts within the pediatric population tend to be developmental and odontogenic in nature.
- Although nonodontogenic cysts of the jaws are relatively uncommon, it is imperative the clinician understand their clinical behavior and management because failure to do so can result in increased patient morbidity.
- The nonodontogenic cysts of the jaws that are most often encountered are the central giant cell granuloma, traumatic bone cavity, aneurysmal bone cyst, nasopalatine duct cyst, and nasolabial cyst.

INTRODUCTION

Nonodontogenic cysts within the jaws are not a common finding in either the adult or pediatric patient population. Shear and Speight[1] conducted a retrospective review of 2616 cysts (in the general population) within the jaws and found 80.1% to be radicular cysts, dentigerous cysts, or odontogenic keratocyst/keratocystic odontogenic tumor. Manor and coworkers[2] found 95 of 322 cysts within the jaws to be in the pediatric (<16) population, with 82% of these being odontogenic. It is well documented that cysts within the pediatric population tend to be developmental and odontogenic in nature.[3,4] Although nonodontogenic cysts of the jaws are relatively uncommon, it is imperative the clinician understand their clinical behavior and management, because failure to do so can result in significantly increased patient morbidity.

The nonodontogenic cysts of the jaws most often encountered are the central giant cell granuloma (CGCG), traumatic bone cyst (TBC), aneurysmal bone cyst (ABC), nasolabial cyst, and nasopalatine duct cyst. This article focuses on the background, clinical findings, radiographic features, histopathologic features, and treatment of these nonodontogenic cysts of the jaws.

CENTRAL GIANT CELL GRANULOMA
Background

This is a benign lesion of unknown cause, possibly from hemorrhage into bone with incomplete healing. It was first described in 1953 by Jaffe who stated that this was a "giant-cell reparative granuloma."[1] The use of the term "reparative" has since been abandoned but may still be seen on older pathology reports, or those written by non–oral and

Disclosure Statement: The authors have nothing to disclose.

[a] Department of Oral and Maxillofacial Surgery, University of Washington, Seattle, WA, USA; [b] Department of Oral and Maxillofacial Surgery, Harborview Medical Center, School of Dentistry, University of Washington, 4West Clinic, 325 9th Avenue, Seattle, WA 98104, USA
* Corresponding author.
E-mail address: dillonj5@uw.edu

Oral Maxillofacial Surg Clin N Am 28 (2016) 31–44
http://dx.doi.org/10.1016/j.coms.2015.08.001

maxillofacial pathologists. The World Health Organization classifies this lesion as a benign idiopathic lesion. It is also considered a reactive lesion that is nonneoplastic in nature, but it can show behavior similar to benign neoplasms.[5] In the 2009 Cochrane review, Suárez-Roa and coworkers[6] described this entity as a rare benign tumor of the jaws with an unknown cause accounting for up to 7% of jaw tumors. Its incidence in the general population is 0.00011% (1 in 900,000).[7] Indeed, Chuong and coworkers[8] first described two variants, nonaggressive and aggressive, with the former being more common. To be classified as aggressive a lesion must have one of the following characteristics: pain, paresthesia, cortical plate perforation, rapid growth, root resorption, or a high rate of recurrence following surgical curettage.[8] Additionally, CGCGs have been shown to be related to cherubism, hyperparathyroidism, neurofibromatosis type 1, and Noonan syndrome.

Clinical Features

This lesion is more common in children and young adults younger than age 30, but can occur at any age.[9] There is a female predilection of 2 to 1. The lesion is more common in the mandible and maxilla, but involvement of other facial bones has been reported.[5] The mandible is affected approximately 70% of the time, with a relatively even distribution in the anterior to posterior regions.[10] Conversely, it is more common in the anterior maxilla, and may cross the midline. Nonaggressive lesions are typically asymptomatic, painless, and slow-growing, and the aggressive lesions present with one or more of the symptoms listed previously. These aggressive lesions are more often found in children and are greater than 5 cm in diameter (**Figs. 1** and **2**).[3]

Radiographic Features

The appearance of these lesions varies greatly, and depends on the criteria that define them as aggressive or nonaggressive. Aggressive lesions often cause displacement of teeth, resorption of roots, and perforation of the cortical plate. They

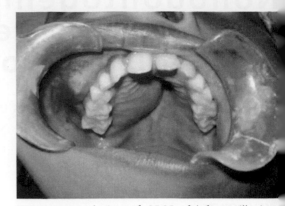

Fig. 2. Intraoral view of CGCG of left maxilla in a 9 year old.

can be unilocular or multilocular, appearing as well-defined, usually with scalloped margins or as an irregular radiolucency. The term "soap bubble" appearance is often used to describe these lesions (see **Figs. 1** and **5**).

Histopathology

A highly cellular, uniform fibroblastic stroma with aggregates of multinucleated giant cells is the diagnostic characteristic of the CGCG. The giant cells may vary in appearance, and extravasated red blood cells are commonly encountered (**Fig. 3**).[4]

Treatment

All patients with an initial diagnosis of CGCG must be investigated further to rule out other diseases, particularly hyperparathyroidism. The first diagnostic adjunct must be a blood test to ascertain serum calcium and parathyroid hormone levels. In true CGCG, these laboratory values are normal. If the calcium and parathyroid hormone levels are elevated, the CGCG diagnosis may represent a brown tumor of hyperparathyroidism. Management of the parathyroid disorder results in resolution of the CGCG. Conventional surgical management of CGCG consists of enucleation and curettage, excision, or en bloc resection with

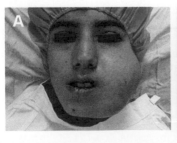
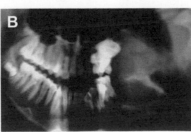

Fig. 1. (A) Locally aggressive CGCG in a 13 year old. (B) Panoramic radiograph. (From Shirani G. Management of a locally invasive central giant cell granuloma (CGCG) of mandible: report of an extraordinary large case. J Craniomaxillofac Surg 2009;37:531; with permission.)

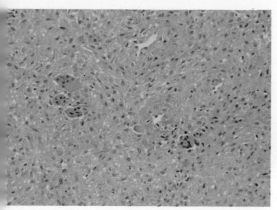

Fig. 3. Histology of CGCG. Note the multinucleated giant cells (H&E stain, original magnification ×100).

or without adjuvant/neoadjuvant medical therapy. Recurrence is common when the lesion is not completely removed. The study by De Lange and coworkers[9] suggests surgery alone is not adequate therapy, citing recurrence rates to be 37.5% in aggressive lesions, whereas Chuong and coworkers[8] found recurrence to be 72%. Tosco and coworkers[10] suggested that en bloc resection is the surgical option with the best predictability, but this treatment is radical and should be avoided in children.[6] Medical therapies include direct intralesional steroid injections, subcutaneous or intranasal calcitonin, and systemic interferon and bisphosphonate therapy, specifically, denosumab, although this is the least studied therapeutic regimen for CGCG (**Fig. 4**).

Calcitonin
Harris,[11] Pogrel,[12] and De Lange and coworkers[9] have studied and reviewed calcitonin therapy and found it to be an effective treatment of CGCG. Calcitonin acts to lower calcium levels by inhibiting bone resorption, counteracting parathyroid hormone. Pogrel[12] reported salmon calcitonin administered as a daily subcutaneous injection to be effective. Intranasal spray (alternating between nostrils to avoid nasal mucosa inflammation) has also been used, but remission rates are lower.[8]

Dosing regimens were based on the treatment of Paget disease, and the duration varied from 19 to 21 months; the treatment continued until there was radiographic evidence of resolution of the lesion.[12] The review by De Lange and coworkers[9] has also found calcitonin to be an effective treatment of CGCG, and dosing was most commonly 100 IU daily subcutaneous injection, or 200 IU when used intranasally. It should be noted that the Food and Drug Administration (FDA) released a drug alert on salmon calcitonin, both the subcutaneous injection and nasal spray forms, in March 2014. This was after a meta-analysis of 21 randomized controlled clinical trials. There was an overall incidence of malignancy of 4.1% compared with placebo-treated patients of 2.9%.[13] Patients should be counseled on the FDA alert and common side effects of nausea, abdominal discomfort, and headache from the use of calcitonin before instituting this form of therapy (**Fig. 5**).

Corticosteroids
The use of intralesional corticosteroid injections is based on the fact that the histopathology of CGCG resembles sarcoidosis, suggesting that because corticosteroid injection is an effective treatment of sarcoidosis, that it would be an effective treatment of CGCG.[11] The technique is direct intralesional injection of a solution of local anesthetic mixed with a corticosteroid, usually triamcinolone. Although the exact dosing and technique may vary, most authors in the review by De Lange and coworkers[9] used triamcinolone, 10 mg/mL, mixed with local anesthetic in a 1:1 ratio, injected once weekly over multiple weeks. Bagheri and coworkers[14] recommend a 50:50 mixture, at 2 mL per 1 cm of lesion visible on panoramic radiograph, injected once weekly over 6 weeks. The literature reports varying rates of success, with Marx and Stern[15] reporting a 65% success rate, whereas multiple case reports show complete success in lesion resolution.[16] The side effects from intralesional steroid–local anesthetic injections are minimal, with the most common adverse event being pain from the injection (despite the use of local anesthetic).

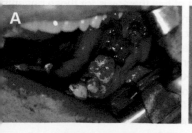
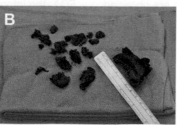

Fig. 4. (A) Traditional enucleation and curettage. Note vascularity of the lesion. (B) CGCG specimen.

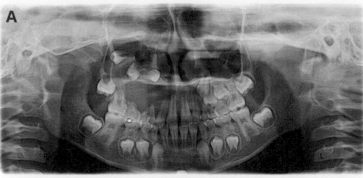

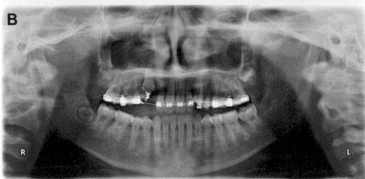

Fig. 5. (A) Panorex of CGCG of patient in Fig. 2. (B) Panorex after treatment of CGCG of the right maxilla with 2 years of subcutaneous calcitonin. Note eruption of permanent teeth and bony fill.

Interferon

The review by De Lange and coworkers[9] also examined the role of interferon in management of the CGCG. Interferon is an antiviral and antiangiogenic agent. This treatment is based on the theory that these lesions may be proliferative vascular lesions. The interferon is thought to suppress the angiogenesis resulting in involution of the lesion. It may also induce the differentiation of mesenchymal stems cells into osteoblasts, leading ultimately to bone formation. The treatment is typically performed in combination with surgery. The usual protocol, per Kaban and coworkers,[17] is that the patient is administered interferon between 48 and 72 hours postoperatively. This is either in the form of interferon alfa-2a or interferon alfa-2b, at a dose of 3 million U/m^2 administered once daily by subcutaneous injection. The mean duration of treatment is 8 months (range, 3.2–16.6). Before commencement of therapy, a baseline complete blood count and liver function tests are obtained. Common side effects are fever or flulike symptoms, rash, nausea, neutropenia, and weight loss. The dosing may need to be adjusted according to the occurrence of side effects, particularly neutropenia. Severe side effects, such as neuropathies and psychosis, may also occur. Side effects must be discussed with the patient and family before commencement of this treatment regimen, and

dose reduction or discontinuation of the drug should be considered in the setting of severe manifestations of side effects. It should be noted that the use of interferon has not been fully validated; however, there are case reports of aggressive CGCG lesions that have had complete remission when interferon usage was combined with surgery.[12,18] The use of interferon may be limited when considering the side effects and alternative available therapies. There are no definitive recommendations regarding patient follow-up, but it is reasonable to follow up every 3 to 6 months with repeat imaging annually.

Bisphosphonates

In June 2013 the FDA approved the use of denosumab (Xgeva, Amgen, Thousand Oaks, CA) to treat adults and some adolescents with giant cell tumor of the bone (GCTB), the term used for these lesions in noncraniofacial bone locations.[19] Per the FDA, the intent of this therapy is for those patients in whom surgery would result in severe morbidity, or if the tumor is considered unresectable. The mechanism of action is based on inhibiting the receptor activator of nuclear factor kappa-B (RANK) and the RANK ligand (RANKL)/osteoprotegerin (OPG) interaction. This results in inhibition of osteoclast activity. RANKL is an essential cytokine for osteoclastogenesis: the survival and activation of osteoclasts. It is essential for healthy bone maintenance. There are three key components in RANKL signaling: (1) the receptor RANK, which is primarily expressed by osteoclasts and mononuclear preosteoclasts; (2) the ligand RANKL, which is a member of the tumor necrosis factor family, is highly expressed by osteoblasts, osteocytes, and periosteal cells; and (3) OPG, a soluble decoy receptor is also expressed by osteoblasts, which acts as a natural negative regulator of RANKL. Denosumab is a fully human monoclonal IgG2 antibody with a high affinity and specificity for RANKL that mimics the effect of OPG, thereby inhibiting the RANK/RANKL interaction.[1] Currently, most of the scientific literature on this class of drug involves the management of GCTB, with FDA approval based on two clinical trials of 305 patients. Waldron and Whitaker in 1995[20] were the first to propose that the CGCG and GCTB belonged to the same spectrum of lesions; however, this is still unclear. As a consequence, therapeutic management of CGCG with denosumab has not been studied extensively.[1] Schreuder and coworkers[7] 2014 published a case report on the use of denosumab for the treatment of a 25-year-old patient with an aggressive CGCG of the maxilla. The patient was administered 120 mg of denosumab via subcutaneous injections for 12 months after failing calcitonin and interferon-2a therapy. They concluded that the use of the bisphosphonate, denosumab, was effective in treating aggressive lesions that did not respond to other modalities of treatment, but that more data are needed before it becomes a mainstay of therapy. Currently, this same academic center has seven patients on denosumab therapy, and preliminary results are promising. The clinician should review the latest literature before considering this new class of medication for CGCG, because the final data from this study are not yet available. The most serious side effect of denosumab is medication-related osteonecrosis of the jaw and osteomyelitis. This has not been seen in the treatment of CGCG to date, but a thorough dental assessment before commencement of this medication regimen is recommended. Other side effects include arthralgia, headache, nausea, fatigue, back pain, and extremity pain. It should not be used by women with reproductive potential, unless they are using highly effective contraception, because there is a risk of fetal harm.

Other therapies

Another agent that works by decreasing RANK, and thus osteoclast activity, is imatinib, a tyrosine kinase inhibitor.[5,21] It is currently used for treatment of leukemia. In 2009, a short communication

by de Lange and coworkers[21] was published on its use in combination with interferon in a patient with Stickler syndrome. It is the senior author's understanding that there are no further data on the usage of imatinib, and it is likely this treatment is no longer in vogue. The reader is reminded to review the latest scientific literature if considering this treatment option. Other therapies, such as human monoclonal antibodies, OPG, and AMG 162, are also currently under investigation.

Summary of Central Giant Cell Granuloma

Clinical
- Benign idiopathic lesion
- Aggressive and nonaggressive
- Usually children and young adults
- Female to male ratio, 2:1
- Mandible > maxilla
- Unilocilar or multilocular radiolucencies

Histopathology
- Highly cellular
- Uniform fibroblastic stroma
- Multinucleated giant cells
- Extravasated red bloods

Treatment
- Enucleation and curettage
- En bloc resection

Adjuvant Medical Therapy
- Calcitonin
- Steroid injections
- Interferon
- Bisphosphonates
- Others

TRAUMATIC BONE CAVITY
Background

TBC is also known by many different names: simple bone cyst, hemorrhagic cyst, intraosseous hematoma, idiopathic bone cyst, extravasation bone cyst, solitary bone cyst, and solitary bone cavity. It also occurs in the long bones, where it is called a simple solitary bone cyst. The nomenclature "cyst" is incorrect, because this lesion does not have an epithelial lining; hence, the term "pseudocyst" is often used. The pathogenesis of TBC is unclear. The most commonly stated cause is hematoma formation within the intramedullary portion of bone secondary to trauma, although patients rarely report a traumatic event. Rather than organizing, the clot breaks down leaving an empty cavity. Other etiologic theories include cystic degeneration of a primary tumor of bone, such as a CGCG; ischemic necrosis of bone/fatty marrow; and possibly a defect in calcium metabolism.[22]

Clinical Features

Teenagers and young adults approximately 10 to 20 years of age are most commonly affected, although TBC can be found in a wide age range and has an equal gender distribution. It is almost exclusively found in the mandible, and has a predilection for the anterior dentate region, but it can be found throughout the mandible. The teeth are usually vital. The lesion is almost always asymptomatic and it is usually an incidental finding on routine dental radiographs where it presents as a solitary area of radiolucency; however, bilateral cases have been reported in the literature. Expansion and pain have been reported, but these are uncommon. The cavity is typically filled with serous or serosanguinous fluid, but may also be completely empty.[23] They are often seen in association with fibro-osseous lesions, such as florid cemento-osseous dysplasia, although the reason for this finding is unclear.[24]

Radiographic Features

TBC is usually a well-defined radiolucency with a sclerotic border. The lesion typically extends between tooth roots with a scalloped appearance, but usually does not cause root resorption or divergence. T2-weighted MRI images show high signal intensity favoring fluid (heme) content (**Figs. 6** and **7**).

Histopathology

Grossly, there is minimal fibrous connective tissue seen within overlying viable bone. Microscopically, there is no evidence of an epithelial component, but a delicate, well-vascularized fibrous connective tissue and hemosiderin may be present. Occasionally giant cells adjacent to the bone surface may be seen.[20]

Treatment

Exploratory surgery, typically performed by directly entering the lesion, confirms the diagnosis and essentially treats the lesion. The area may be curetted to encourage bleeding, and then closed primarily. Subsequent organization of the clot leads to complete bony healing, although cases of recurrence have been reported. Hatakeyama and coworkers[22] discussed endoscopy as a useful method for an unusual condylar head TBC lesion, citing the technique as minimally invasive and with low morbidity (**Fig. 8**).

Summary of Traumatic Bone Cavity

Clinical
- Pseudocyst with no epithelial lining
- Teenagers/young adults
- Male to female ratio, 1:1
- Almost exclusive to mandible
- Well-defined radiolucency with sclerotic borders

Histopathology
- Minimal fibrous connective tissue
- No evidence of an epithelial component
- Delicate, well-vascularized fibrous connective tissue and hemosiderin
- Occasional giant cells

Treatment
- Enucleation and curettage

ANEURYSMAL BONE CYST
Background

ABC is an uncommon lesion of the jaws that is more commonly present in long bones. Similar to TBC, the nomenclature is confusing because this is a pseudocyst (it has no epithelial lining). It was first described by Jaffe and Lichtenstein in 1942.[25,26] The World Health Organization describes this as an expansile, multilocular, osteolytic lesion, with blood-filled spaces separated by

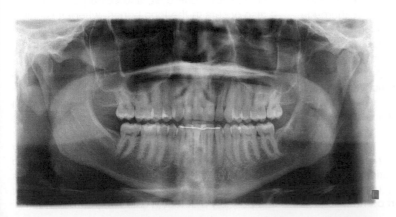

Fig. 6. Panorex of a traumatic bone cavity of the left mandibular ramus.

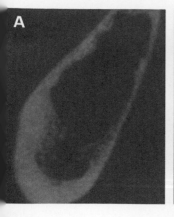
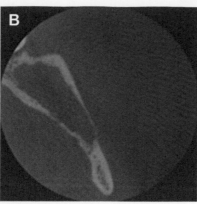

Fig. 7. (*A*) Computed tomography (CT) scan of traumatic bone cavity of left mandible: coronal view. (*B*) CT scan of traumatic bone cavity of left mandible: axial view.

fibrous septa-containing osteoclast-type giant cells and reactive bone.[27] Sun and coworkers found this lesion to be documented only 92 times, whereas the review by Shear and Speight only found these to occur 0.4% of the time.[28,29] The cause is ultimately unknown, with multiple theories proposed, ranging from vascular abnormalities leading to high-pressure hemorrhage, reactive cause, and possible genetic predisposition.[30,31] The review by Sun and coworkers[28] did not find any history of trauma associated with these lesions, but this has also been suggested as a possible cause.

Clinical Features

ABC is more common in patients younger than 30, but it can occur at any age. Although epidemiologic data are lacking, most studies find no gender predilection.[24,32,33] ABC is found more often in the mandible than the maxilla, with the posterior regions, in particular the ramus and posterior body, accounting for 51.7% of lesions. Reports of ABC presenting in the zygoma, sphenoid, ethmoid, temporal, and occipital bones are well documented. Commonly, ABC presents as painless swelling. There is no associated thrill or bruit on auscultation. Aspiration may yield blood. Teeth

remain vital, although displacement, loosening, and resorption of teeth may be seen.[25] Pain has been reported usually when the lesion grows rapidly. Rarely patients may report paresthesia or malocclusion (**Fig. 9**).

Radiographic Features

These can be similar to CGCG, with irregular and expansile borders that can vary in appearance. They may be unilocular or multilocular in nature, with or without well-defined borders. Root resorption and cortical plate perforation may be seen. When present as a multilocular lesion, as with CGCG, these lesions are often described as having a "soap bubble" appearance. On MRI, T2-weighted imaging has high signal intensity and reveals fluid-fluid levels caused by blood cell sedimentation (**Figs. 10** and **11**).[25]

Histopathology

These entities are pseudocysts, because there is no epithelial lining. One variant of ABC is the

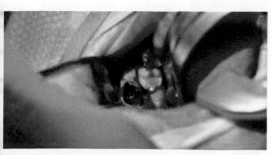

Fig. 8. Intraoral approach to traumatic bone cavity.

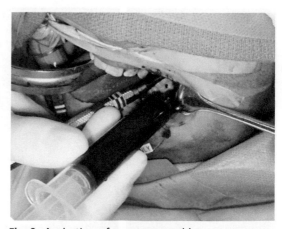

Fig. 9. Aspiration of an aneurysmal bone cyst.

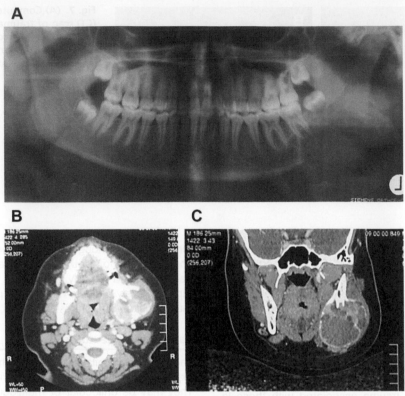

Fig. 10. *A*) Panorex of an aneurysmal bone cyst of the left mandible. (*B*) Aneurysmal bone cyst of the left mandible. Axial view CT with soft tissue window. (*C*) Aneurysmal bone cyst of the left mandible. Coronal view CT with bone window.

classic, or vascular, type. This is multilocular, well circumscribed, with blood-filled cavities, lined by macrophages and osteoclast-like giant cells.[25] The second variant is the solid type, with solid gray-white tissue, abundant with fibroblastic, osteoid, and calcifying fibromyxoid tissue. The third variant is a combination of the two, and is usually the most commonly encountered form of ABC (**Fig. 12**).[22,24]

Treatment

Classic treatment is thorough curettage or resection. Variable rates of recurrence have been

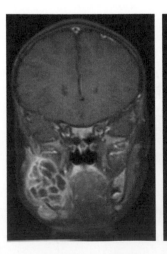

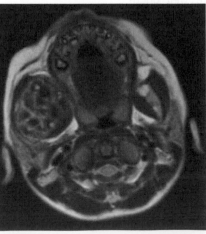

Fig. 11. MRI of an aneurysmal bone cyst of the right mandible. (*From* Ariffin S, Yunus N. Aneurysmal bone cyst of the mandible: a case report. Pediatr Dent J 2014;24(3):181; with permission.)

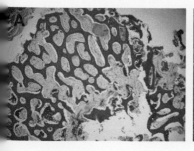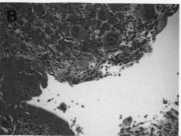

Fig. 12. (*A*) Histopathologic slide of aneurysmal bone cyst; low power (H&E stains, original magnification ×10). (*B*) Histopathologic slide of aneurysmal bone cyst; high power. Note multinucleated giant cells (H&E stains, original magnification ×40).

reported, with higher rates associated with curettage.[24] It has been suggested that because of intraoperative hemorrhage, adequate removal is difficult to achieve, especially in cases of large and aggressive lesions. En bloc resection has the lowest chance of recurrence, but is associated with increased morbidity.[34] Other treatments that have been suggested as adjuncts to surgery include cryotherapy, steroids, calcitonin, and embolization. Embolization has been used successfully in the ABC cases of long bones but there is limited evidence on its use within the head and neck. Kumar and coworkers[34] reported a series of three cases in which recurrent, large, and aggressive lesions were treated using embolization via n-butyl cyanoacrylate glue. At 4 months postembolization, there was no evidence of bone formation, and all the patients ultimately underwent en bloc resection and reconstruction with minimal intraoperative blood loss. The conclusions were that surgical curettage, or resection, remains the standard of therapy, but embolization may prove to be a useful adjuvant therapy for a relatively bloodless surgical field (**Figs. 13–15**).[31]

Summary of Aneurysmal Bone Cyst

Clinical
- Pseudocyst with no epithelial lining
- Patients usually younger than 30
- Male to female ratio, 1:1
- Mandible >maxilla
- Unilocular or multilocular radiolucency

Histopathology
- 3 types: classic (vascular), solid, mixed
- Multilocular, well circumscribed with blood-filled cavities, lined by macrophages and osteoclast-like giant cells
- Solid type: solid gray-white tissue, abundant with fibroblastic, osteoid, and calcifying fibromyxoid tissue
- Mixed type: most common

Treatment
- Enucleation and curettage
- En bloc resection

NASOPALATINE DUCT CYST
Background

This is also called the incisive canal cyst or median palatine cyst when located more posteriorly in the palate. This is the most common nonodontogenic cyst of the oral cavity. It has been found to occur in 2.2% to 11.6% of the population, or 1 in every 100 persons.[35] The nasopalatine canal forms secondary to fusion of the left and right palatine processes to the premaxilla. The anatomic exit of the canal lies slightly posterior to the incisive papilla. The nasopalatine duct typically degenerates in humans, but epithelial remnants remain, with the potential for cystic enlargement. Other structures found within the canal include the nasopalatine nerve, and branches of the descending palatine and sphenopalatine arteries.

The most likely cause of this cyst is from persistence of the epithelial remnants following duct degeneration.[36] However, the precise stimulus to cystic formation is unclear. Various theories proposed include trauma (eg, removable dentures, treatment with dental implants), bacterial infection,

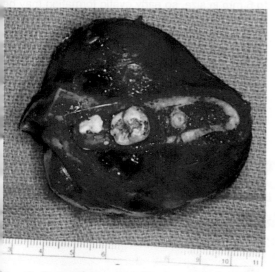

Fig. 13. Resected aneurysmal bone cyst specimen.

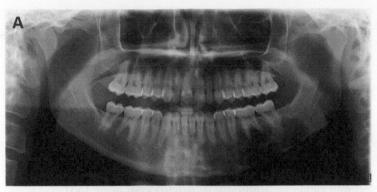

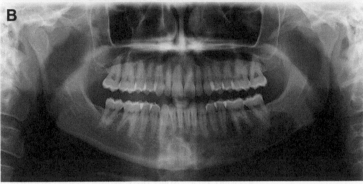

Fig. 14. (A) Preoperative panorex of aneurysmal bone cyst treated by enucleation and curettage. (B) A 4-month postoperative panorex of aneurysmal bone cyst treated by enucleation and curettage.

or the presence of mucus glands within the epithelium causing mucus retention.

Clinical Features

This lesion has a male predilection of 3:1.[33,35,37] It is most common in the fourth to sixth decades, but can occur at any age. In the review by Swanson and coworkers[36] of 334 cases, the median age was 42.5. Typically it is found incidentally on dental radiographs; however, pain, upper lip swelling, or drainage can occur, especially if the cyst is secondarily infected. Sinus formation and drainage at the palatine papilla may be seen. The rate of symptomatic lesions varies throughout the literature and does not seem to follow any predictable patterns, such as age or size.[32]

Radiographic Features

Typically a well-circumscribed, round, ovoid, or heart-shaped radiolucency near the maxillary incisors is found radiographically. It can sometimes be difficult to differentiate this lesion from other lesions, or simply normal anatomic variants. The nasopalatine duct cysts range in size from several millimeters to centimeters. The average size is 1.5 cm. Of note, the incisive foramen can be up to 6 mm in size, so early cystic formation may be difficult to detect. When the lesion is larger than 1 cm, other lesions, such as radicular cysts or keratocystic odontogenic tumors, may be initial considerations in the differential diagnosis.[32,33] The lamina dura of associated teeth is intact, but larger lesions can cause root divergence and resorption. Cone beam computed tomography

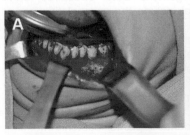

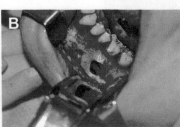

Fig. 15. (A) ABC. Note blue hue of the lesion before enucleation and curettage. (B) ABC. Note sparse soft tissue and inferior alveolar nerve.

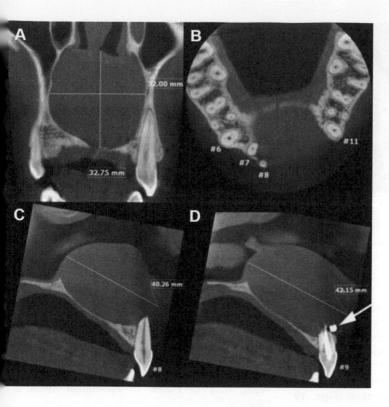

Fig. 16. (*A–D*) Cone beam CT of a large nasopalatine duct cyst. (*From* Suter V, Sendi P, Reichart P, et al. The nasopalatine duct cyst: an analysis of the relation between clinical symptoms, cyst dimensions, and involvement of neighboring anatomic structures using cone beam computed tomography. J Oral Maxillofac Surg 2011;69(10):2597, 2598; with permission.)

(CT) or medical-grade CT can be useful in analyzing these lesions (**Figs. 16** and **17**).

Histopathology

This may vary depending on where the sample is derived. Superiorly (toward the nasal cavity), the likely histology is of respiratory epithelium, pseudostratified columnar epithelium with or without goblets cells, whereas inferiorly (toward the oral cavity) it is more likely to be stratified squamous epithelium. A combination of the two can be found.[32–34,38] Additionally, nerves, arteries, veins, minor salivary glands, and small islands of cartilage may be found. If the cyst had been infected, the specimen may contain inflammatory cells (**Fig. 18**).

Treatment

Treatment typically depends on the presenting symptoms. Surgical excision and curettage is adequate therapy. Access may be palatal, or a combination of labial and palatal, depending on the size and location of the nasopalatine duct cyst. The review by Swanson and coworkers[36] of

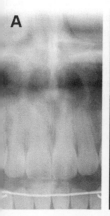
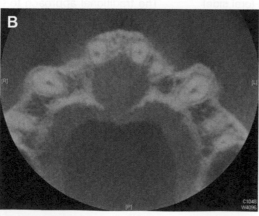

Fig. 17. (*A*) Nasopalatine duct cyst. Note classic heart-shaped radiolucency of the nasopalatine duct cyst. (*B*) Nasopalatine duct cyst; CT axial view, bone window.

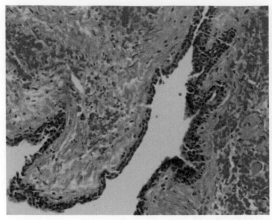

Fig. 18. High-power histology of a nasopalatine duct cyst. Note respiratory epithelium (original magnification ×40).

334 cases showed a recurrence rate of only 2%. Common complications of treatment can include damage to the nasal floor, oroantral ororonasal communication or fistula, and possible damage to adjacent teeth. In cases of larger lesions, marsupialization may be indicated to decrease the size of the cyst before enucleation (**Figs. 19 and 20**).[34]

Summary of Nasopalatine Duct Cyst

Clinical
- Most common nonodontogenic cyst
- Male to female ratio, 3:1
- Fourth to fifth decade, but can be found in young patients
- Usually incidental finding
- Well-circumscribed, round, ovoid, or heart-shaped radiolucency near the maxillary incisors

Histopathology
- Pseudostratified columnar epithelium, with or without goblets cells (nasal side)
- Stratified squamous epithelium (oral side)

Treatment
- Surgical excision and curettage

NASOLABIAL CYST
Background

This is a rare developmental cyst, comprising only 0.7% of all jaw cysts.[39,40] It occurs in the upper lip, lateral of midline, or near the junction of the lateral and canine tooth. One theory maintains that the nasolabial cyst arises from the entrapped epithelial remnants along the fusion line of the maxillary medial and lateral nasal processes during embryogenesis. Another theory suggests it arises from ectopic epithelium of the nasolacrimal duct.[37]

Clinical Features

These include swelling of the upper lip, elevation of the ala of the nose, obliteration of the vestibule, and elevation of the mucosa of the nasal vestibule. If large, it can obstruct the nasal aperture and interfere with denture seating, and a common complaint from patients is the onset of a facial deformity.[41] It is usually asymptomatic, unless it becomes secondarily infected. It is more commonly found in adults in the fourth and fifth decade of life, but can be found in children, and has a distinct female predilection of nearly 4:1. Also, 10% of cases of nasolabial cysts are bilateral.[42]

Radiographic Features

The nasolabial cyst is not visualized with traditional plain film radiographs because they are soft tissue lesions. Cone beam CT, traditional CT, or MRI show a soft tissue mass of varying size that is usually well-demarcated.

Histopathology

A cystic structure lined by pseudostratified columnar epithelium is most commonly seen, but cuboidal epithelium can occasionally be found.[37]

Treatment

The traditional approach to this lesion is surgical excision via an intraoral/sublabial approach. The surgeon must be aware of the close proximity to

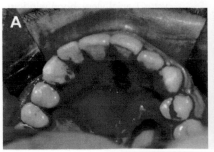

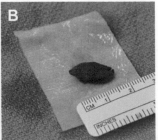

Fig. 19. (*A*) Enucleation and curettage of a nasopalatine duct cyst. (*B*) Specimen of nasopalatine duct cyst.

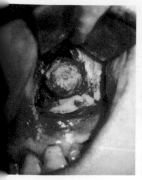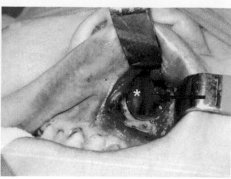

Fig. 20. Enucleation and curettage of nasolabial cyst via an intraoral approach. *Arrow,* inferior turbinate; *, nasal septum. (*From* Yuen H, Julian C, Samuel C. Nasolabial cysts: clinical features, diagnosis, and treatment. Br J Oral Maxillofac Surg 2007;45(4):295; with permission.)

the nasal mucosa and nasal floor. This may require sacrifice of the nasal mucosa to ensure complete removal, with repair of an oronasal fistula during or following surgical treatment of the cyst. Other approaches include endoscopic marsupialization via a transnasal approach. Chao and coworkers[39] reviewed 57 cases and compared the sublabial approach with the endoscopic approach. The endoscopic approach had shorter surgery times, lower hospitalization rates, and lower medical costs, but was no more effective because no differences in rates of recurrence were seen (see **Fig. 19**).

Summary of Nasolabial Cyst

Clinical
- Development cyst
- Asymptomatic
- Fourth and fifth decade, but can be found in young patients
- Male to female ratio, 4:1
- Upper lip, lateral of midline
- Swelling, facial deformity
- 10% bilateral

Histopathology
- Pseudostratified columnar epithelium

Treatment
- Surgical excision via intraoral approach usually

REFERENCES

1. Shear M, Speight PM. Cysts of the oral and maxillofacial regions. Oral Surg Oral Med Oral Pathol Oral Radiol Endod 2007;43:1049.
2. Manor E, Kachko L, Puterman MB, et al. Cystic lesions of the jaws: a clinicopathological study of 322 cases and review of the literature. Int J Med Sci 2012;9(1):20–6.
3. Bodner L. Cystic lesions of the jaws in children. Int J Pediatr Otorhinolaryngol 2002;62:25–9.
4. Iatrou I, Theologie-Lygidakis N, Leventis M. Intraosseous cystic lesions of the jaws in children: a retrospective analysis of 47 consecutive cases. Oral Surg Oral Med Oral Pathol Oral Radiol Endod 2009;107:485–92.
5. Gianluca N, Lorè B, Mariani G. Central giant cell granuloma of the jaws. J Craniofac Surg 2010;21: 383–6.
6. Suárez-Roa Mde L, Reveiz L, Ruíz-Godoy Rivera LM, et al. Interventions for central giant cell granuloma (CGCG) of the jaws. Cochrane Database Syst Rev 2009;(4):CD007404.
7. Schreuder W, Coumou A, Kessler P, et al. Alternative pharmacologic therapy for aggressive central giant cell granuloma: denosumab. J Oral Maxillofac Surg 2014;72(7):1301–9.
8. Chuong R, Kaban LB, Kozakewich H, et al. Central giant cell lesions of the jaws: a clinicopathologic study. J Oral Maxillofac Surg 1986;44(9):714–8.
9. de Lange J, van den Akker HP, van den Berg H. Central giant cell granuloma of the jaw: a review of the literature with emphasis on therapy options. Oral Surg Oral Med Oral Pathol Oral Radiol Endod 2007;104(5):603–15.
10. Tosco P, Tanteri G, Iaquinta C, et al. Surgical treatment and reconstruction for central giant cell granuloma of the jaws: a review of 18 cases. J Craniomaxillofac Surg 2009;37(7):380–7.
11. Harris M. Central giant cell granulomas of the jaws regress with calcitonin therapy. Br J Oral Maxillofac Surg 1993;31(2):89–94.
12. Pogrel M. Calcitonin therapy for central giant cell granuloma. J Craniomaxillofac Surg 2003;61(6): 649–53.
13. Miacalcin (calcitonin-salmon) Injection and Nasal Spray. Miacalcin (calcitonin-salmon) Injection and Nasal Spray. Ed. FDA. US Food and Drug Administration, Mar. 2014. Web. 16 May 2015. Available at: http://www.accessdata.fda.gov/scripts/cder/drugsatfda/index.cfm.
14. Bagheri S, Bell B, Khan H. The Central giant cell granuloma. Current therapy in oral and maxillofacial

surgery. St. Louis, (MO): Elsevier Saunders; 2012. p. 410–3.

15. Marx R, Stern D. A rationale for diagnosis. Oral and Maxillofacial Pathology. Chicago 2003;783–79.

16. Ferretti C, Muthray E. Management of central giant cell granuloma of mandible using intralesional corticosteroids: case report and review of literature. J Oral Maxillofac Surg 2011;69(11):2824–9.

17. Kaban L, Troulis M, Ebb D, et al. Antiangiogenic therapy with interferon alpha for giant cell lesions of the jaws. J Oral Maxillofac Surg 2002;60(10): 1103–11.

18. Kaban L, Troulis M, Ebb D, et al. Adjuvant antiangiogenic therapy for giant cell tumors of the jaws. J Oral Maxillofac Surg 2007;65(10):2018–24.

19. Pazdur R. FDA approval for dunosumab. National Cancer Institute. National Institutes of Health; 2013. Web. 29 Apr. 2015. Available at: http://www.cancer.gov/about-cancer/treatment/drugs/fda-denosumab.

20. Vered M, Buchner A, Dayan D. Central giant cell granuloma of the jawbones – new insights into molecular biology with clinical implications on treatment approaches. Histol Histopathol 2008;23:1151–60.

21. de Lange J, Rick R, Rijn V, et al. Regression of central giant cell granuloma by a combination of imatinib and interferon: a case report. Br J Oral Maxillofac Surg 2009;47:59–61.

22. Hatakeyama D, Tamaoki N, Iida K, et al. Simple bone cyst of the mandibular condyle in a child: report of a case. J Oral Maxillofac Surg 2012;70(9):2118–23.

23. Barnes L, Eveson JW, Reichert P, et al. World Health Organization classification of tumors: pathology and genetics of head and neck tumors. Lyon (France): IARC Press; 2005. p. 327.

24. Wakasa T, Kawai N, Aiga H, et al. Management of florid cemento-osseous dysplasia of the mandible producing solitary bone cyst: report of a case. J Oral Maxillofac Surg 2002;60(7):832–5.

25. Motamedi M, Behroozian A, Aziz T, et al. Assessment of 120 maxillofacial aneurysmal bone cysts: a nationwide quest to understand this enigma. J Oral Maxillofac Surg 2014;72:1523–30.

26. Jaffe H, Lichtenstein L. Solitary unicameral bone cyst with emphasis on the roentgen picture, the pathologic appearance and the pathogenesis. Arch Surg 1942;44(6):1004–25.

27. Barnes L, Eveson JW, Reichert P, et al. World Health Organization classification of tumors: pathology and genetics of head and neck tumors. Lyon (France): IARC Press; 2005. p. 326.

28. Sun Z, Zhao Y, Yang R, et al. Aneurysmal bone cysts of the jaws: analysis of 17 cases. J Oral Maxillofac Surg 2010;68(9):2122–8.

29. Shear M, Speight PM. Cysts of the oral and maxillofacial regions. Oral Surg Oral Med Oral Pathol Oral Radiol Endod 2007;43:543.

30. Biesecker J, Marcove R, Huvos A, et al. Aneurysmal bone cysts: a clinicopathologic study of 66 cases. Cancer 1970;26:615.

31. Panoutsakopoulos G, Pandis N, Kyriazoglou I, et al. Recurrent (16;17)(q22;p13) in aneurysmal bone cysts. Genes Chromosomes Cancer 1999;26:265.

32. Ariffin S, Yunus N. Aneurysmal bone cyst of the mandible: a case report. Pediatr Dent J 2014; 24(3):178–83.

33. Kaffe I, Naor H, Calderon S, et al. Radiological and clinical features of aneurysmal bone cyst of the jaws. DentomaxillofacRadiol 1999;28:167.

34. Kumar V, Malik N, Kumar D. Treatment of large recurrent aneurysmal bone cysts of mandible: transosseous intralesional embolization as an adjunct to resection. Int J Oral Maxillofac Surg 2009;38(6): 671–6.

35. Suter V, Sendi P, Reichart P, et al. Expansive nasopalatine duct cysts with nasal involvement mimicking apical lesions of endodontic origin: a report of two cases. J Endod 2011;37(9):1320–6.

36. Swanson K, Kaugars G, Gunsolley J. Nasopalatine duct cyst: an analysis of 334 cases. J Oral Maxillofac Surg 1991;49(3):268–71.

37. Allard R, Van Der Kwast W, Van der Waal I. Nasopalatine duct cyst: review of the literature and report of 22 cases. Int J Oral Surg 1981;10(6):447–61.

38. Bodin I, Isacsson G, Julin P. Cysts of the nasopalatine duct. Int J Oral Maxillofac Surg 1986;15(6): 696–706, 7.

39. Chao W, Huang C, Chang P, et al. Management of nasolabial cysts by transnasal endoscopic marsupialization. Arch Otolaryngol Head Neck Surg 2009; 135:932–5.

40. el-Din K, el-Hamd AA. Nasolabial cyst: a report of eight cases and a review of the literature. J Laryngol Otol 1999;113:747–9.

41. Yuen H, Julian C, Samuel C. Nasolabial cysts: clinical features, diagnosis, and treatment. Br J Oral Maxillofac Surg 2007;45(4):293–7.

42. Neville BW. Developmental defects of the oral and maxillofacial region. Oral and maxillofacial pathology. St Louis (MO): Saunders/Elsevier; 2009. p. 27–8.

Pediatric Odontogenic Tumors

Joshua M. Abrahams, DMD[a,b,*], Shawn A. McClure, DMD, MD, FACS[a]

KEYWORDS

- Odontogenic tumor • Ameloblastoma • Odontoma • Jaws • Mandible • Maxilla

KEY POINTS

- Pediatric odontogenic tumors are mostly benign lesions, and are categorized based on their cells and tissues of origin.
- They typically occur in the posterior mandible region and are often associated with an impacted tooth.
- Most odontogenic tumors are amenable to simple enucleation and curettage; however, more aggressive or recurrent lesions may require radical surgery with appropriate reconstruction.
- Fear of disfigurement or psychosocial reasoning often influences surgeons to perform conservative treatment on children; however, serious consequences can occur, which include recurrence or malignant transformation of the tumor.

INTRODUCTION

Odontogenic tumors are rare tumors that affect patients in the maxillofacial region. These tumors can be varied in their presenting symptoms, overall growth rate and magnitude, and degree of tissue destruction. Many odontogenic tumors present with minimal symptoms, and are discovered only incidentally on radiographic examination.

If the lesion is symptomatic, patients typically present with rapid growth and expansion of their jaws. Cosmetic appearance may be altered with facial asymmetry, and there may be displacement and loosening of teeth in the affected area. Paresthesia of the inferior alveolar nerve is an unusual symptom because of the benign nature of these odontogenic tumors. If the inferior alveolar nerve is affected, this could indicate a long-standing lesion, or a malignant process.

Most of these tumors are benign and easily amenable to extirpative surgery, such as enucleation and curettage. More aggressive benign lesions, as well as malignant tumors, require radical ablative surgery with appropriate immediate or delayed reconstruction. Although benign, if not treated appropriately, more aggressive odontogenic tumors will recur in anatomic locations of the head and neck that may be unresectable, thereby becoming life threatening because of airway compromise or cranial base involvement.[1]

On a histologic level, odontogenic tumors are divided into 3 categories: epithelial, mesenchymal, and mixed epithelial and mesenchymal odontogenic tumors. Each category is defined based on the tissue from which the tumors arise.

Overall, oral and maxillofacial tumors in the pediatric population are rare. Studies are retrospective in nature, and usually combine multiple surgeon and institutional experiences. Overwhelmingly, these tumors are benign in most case series.[2] Soft tissue tumors, such as hemangiomas, papillomas, and lymphangiomas, make up close to 70% of all the head and neck tumors in the pediatric population.[3] Pediatric odontogenic

Financial disclosures: None.
[a] Department of Oral and Maxillofacial Surgery, Broward Health Medical Center, Nova Southeastern University College of Dental Medicine, 3200 S. University Dr. Ft. Lauderdale, FL 33328, USA; [b] Long Island Oral and Maxillofacial Surgery, 134 Mineola Blvd. Mineola, New York 11501, USA
* Corresponding author.
E-mail address: abrahamsdmd@gmail.com

Oral Maxillofacial Surg Clin N Am 28 (2016) 45–58
http://dx.doi.org/10.1016/j.coms.2015.08.003
1042-3699/16/$ – see front matter © 2016 Elsevier Inc. All rights reserved.

tumors consist of only one-third of the tumors seen in the maxillofacial region. The most common lesions are odontoma, ameloblastoma, and the keratocystic odontogenic tumor (KCOT).

Most literature reviews agree that the preponderance of development of these odontogenic tumors occurs in the pediatric population after the age of 6 years. It is during this time of secondary tooth development that the dental crown is being formed. Alteration in these particular cells can lead to the formation of odontogenic tumors.

EPITHELIAL ODONTOGENIC TUMORS

Odontogenic tumors of this category usually originate from the epithelial cells of tooth development. As the secondary teeth begin to develop and grow, cells from the rest of the dental lamina, developing enamel organ, epithelial lining of odontogenic cysts, and the basilar epithelial cells of the gingival surface epithelium, can be altered in their development.[4] Most of these tumors occurring in the pediatric population are ameloblastomas. KCOTs are also seen frequently in syndromic children (eg, basal cell nevus syndrome).

Ameloblastoma

Epidemiology
Ameloblastoma is the most common aggressive benign tumor of the mandible and maxilla. However, its occurrence in the pediatric population is rare. Most case series and retrospective reviews across multiple institutions report that 10% to 15% of cases present in the pediatric age group.[5] Ameloblastomas are classified into 3 major histologic subtypes: solid or multicystic, unicystic, and peripheral.

Unlike adult ameloblastomas, the pediatric population has a higher percentage of unicystic ameloblastomas. Most involve unerupted teeth, because it is thought that the lesions are produced de novo by neoplastic transformation of the non-neoplastic cyst lining.[4] Ackerman, and colleagues[6] described 3 histologic subtypes for the unicystic ameloblastoma. Type 1 and 2 have epithelium with no invasion into the fibrous cyst wall. Type 3 invades into the cyst wall either in a follicular or plexiform pattern, thereby having the capacity to invade adjacent bone (**Fig. 1**). Type 3 should be considered as aggressive a lesion as the conventional ameloblastoma.

The unicystic ameloblastoma mimics a dentigerous cyst clinically and radiographically, and therefore simple enucleation is often the treatment that is recommended and performed. The pathologic diagnosis of unicystic ameloblastoma is often surprising, with the expectation of a

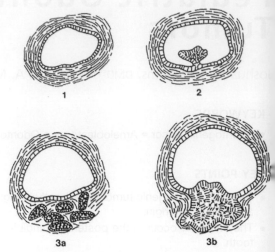

Fig. 1. Histologic subtypes: 1 and 2. Type 1 and 2 show no invasion into the fibrous cyst wall. 3. Type 3 shows invasion into the cystic wall in type 3a (follicular) or type 3b (plexiform) pattern. (*From* Ackermann GL, Altini M, Shear M. The unicystic ameloblastoma: a clinicopathological study of 57 cases. J Oral Pathol 1988;17:541; with permission.)

dentigerous cyst, leading the surgeon to question whether further treatment is indicated.[7]

Location
- Similar to adults, almost all occur in the body and angle of the mandible
- Location in the maxilla is very rare in the pediatric population; single case reports are noted in the literature

Symptoms
- Slow-growing facial deformity (**Fig. 2**)
- Tooth mobility and buccal expansion seen intraorally
- Complaints of pain and paresthesia are rare

Radiographic features
- Most have a unicystic appearance (**Fig. 3**)
  - Even solid ameloblastomas can appear unicystic on radiographs in pediatric patients

Treatment
Treatment of pediatric ameloblastoma can be controversial. As stated earlier, most pediatric ameloblastomas appear to be dentigerous cysts on clinical and radiographic examination. The diagnosis of unicystic ameloblastoma after enucleation can lead practitioners to undertreat patients in this population. Fearing the potential interruption of facial growth and loss of function, treating physicians have patients undergo the

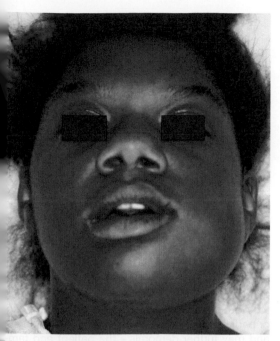

Fig. 2. A 14-year-old African American girl showing left-sided facial swelling approximately 1 year in duration.

most minimal and conservative surgery, which may lead to multiple recurrences. **Fig. 4** details surgical treatment of a pediatric patient diagnosed with an ameloblastoma.

With a diagnosis of a conventional or Ackerman type 3 ameloblastoma, the treatment of choice should be resection with at least 1.0-cm to 1.5-cm margins of normal bone (**Fig. 5**). If the ameloblastoma is contained within the maxilla, surgical resection should be recommended. Thin cortical bone and large marrow spaces of the maxilla may allow the tumor to spread to the orbit and skull base, and seed within the pterygoid muscles. Once this occurs, surgical cure becomes increasingly difficult. Because the tumor is fairly radioinsensitive, radiation therapy is of limited use.

Most pediatric ameloblastomas occur in the mandible. Each patient diagnosed with ameloblastoma requires an individualized treatment plan, because not all tumors can be treated in a similar fashion. The factors to consider include the location, size, and perforation of existing cortices in order to adequately plan the surgical resection and reconstruction.

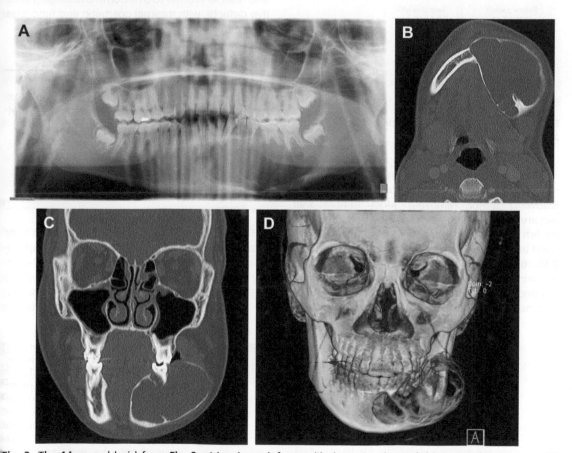

Fig. 3. The 14-year-old girl from **Fig. 2** with a large left mandibular unicystic ameloblastoma. (*A*) Panorex. (*B*) Axial computed tomography (CT) scan. (*C*) Coronal CT scan. (*D*) Three-dimensional reconstruction.

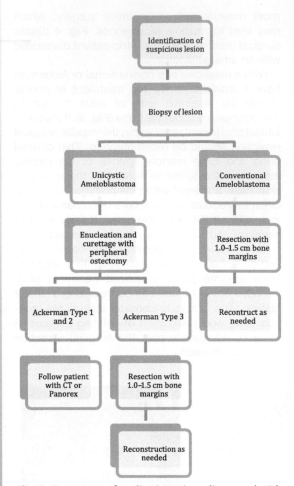

Fig. 4. Treatment of pediatric patient diagnosed with ameloblastoma.

Some investigators maintain that rapid bone regeneration occurs if the periosteum is left intact following tumor removal.[3] Most tumors that require resection do not allow the periosteum to be left intact. In most cases, the periosteum is used as a margin covering the cortical perforation (**Fig. 6**). This ablative defect is often complex, requiring both bony and soft tissue reconstruction.

Adequate reconstruction and the avoidance of psychosocial effects in pediatric patients can

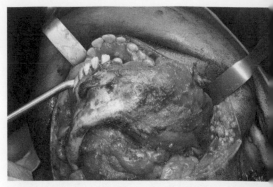

Fig. 6. Cortical perforation of mandible required the periosteum to be sacrificed as a margin (anatomic layer).

be demanding. There is a tendency to treat childhood ameloblastomas conservatively. Immediate microvascular reconstruction has been designed to overcome the limitations of other flaps. Local or pedicled flaps may require multiple procedures and may further demoralize the patient and family.[8] Overall, free tissue transfer in children is safe and reliable in order to overcome challenging ablative defects, with minimal cosmetic and functional deformity in pediatric patients.

Malignant Ameloblastoma

Epidemiology
Despite its benign histologic appearance, approximately 2% of ameloblastomas metastasize.[9] Metastatic lesions have been identified in:

- Lungs (most common)
- Cervical nodes
- Vertebrae
- Kidneys
- Heart

The increased incidence of metastasis has been attributed to large, long-standing tumors, inappropriately treated ameloblastomas, and multiple surgeries within the same anatomic area. Because the metastatic deposits are histologically similar to the primary ameloblastoma, and hence

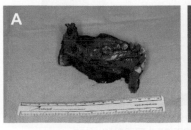
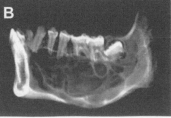

Fig. 5. (*A*) Resection of the left mandibular unicystic ameloblastoma included a 1.0-cm to 1.5-cm margin of normal bone. A reconstruction plate was applied to maintain the anatomic shape and function of the mandible. (*B*) Intraoperative radiograph of the specimen shows the margins free of tumor.

nsensitive to radiation, surgery is recommended for removal of the metastatic deposits.

Ameloblastic Carcinoma

Epidemiology

Ameloblastic carcinoma is a rare malignant odontogenic tumor. A review of the literature has only identified 18 pediatric cases from 1932 to 2012.[10] Unlike adult tumors, these pediatric cases are evenly diagnosed in the maxilla and mandible.

- Primary type: develops de novo
- Secondary type:
  - Intraosseous ameloblastoma
  - Peripheral ameloblastoma

Symptoms

- Expansion of affected jaw with rapid tumor growth
- Tooth mobility, pain, paresthesia
- Tumor extension into surrounding soft tissues

Treatment

Once diagnosed, the patient should undergo a total-body staging work-up, which includes computed tomography of the head, neck, and chest. Surgery with therapeutic neck dissection is recommednded.[11] Because of the paucity of tumors that have been diagnosed and treated, their radiosensitivity and the role of chemotherapy have not yet been elucidated.[11]

Keratocystic Odontogenic Tumor

Epidemiology

Thought to have arisen from the dental lamina, the term odontogenic keratocyst (OKC) was introduced in 1956 by Philipsen.[12] This term was used to describe a benign, but locally destructive, odontogenic cyst. Once treated as a benign entity, the recurrence rate was unacceptably high after simple enucleation. Contributing to the recurrence is a thin, friable cystic lining and daughter cysts, entrenched beyond the visible margin of the cyst. In addition, residual tumor or daughter cysts between the superior periphery of the cyst and oral mucosa are known to be a possible cause of recurrence. Although various methods of surgical removal have been investigated, recurrence rates were encountered with each proposed treatment modality.

On histology, the odontogenic keratocyst is lined by orthokeratinized or parakeratinized epithelium. In general, the parakeratinized type is the more aggressive and destructive of the two forms. Because of its aggressive nature, high recurrence rates, and the presence of tumor markers (proliferating cell nuclear antigen), the

World Health Organization (WHO) renamed the lesion KCOT in 2005.[13]

KCOT in the pediatric population is seen mostly in syndromic patients; more specifically, basal cell nevus syndrome (BCNS). BCNS is an autosomal dominant disorder with variable penetrance, based on the *Patched* gene (*PCTH1*) on chromosome 9q. It is thought to hold *Smoothened* (*SMO*), a transmembrane protein in an inactive state, thus inhibiting signaling to downstream genes.[14]

Classically, children affected with this disorder have multiple basal cell carcinomas (BCCs), frontal bossing, coarse facial features, bifid ribs, palmar and plantar pitting, calcification of the falx cerebri, and multiple KCOTs (**Fig. 7**). Recurrent BCCs are generally on non–sun-exposed areas of the body so exposure to ultraviolet light should be limited in these individuals. **Box 1** shows other frequent features of the syndrome.

Location

- From 60% to 80% involve the posterior mandible and ascending ramus

Symptoms

- Expands through marrow spaces of the bone, because of proteolytic enzymes along the tumor capsule
- Rarely has buccal expansion

Radiographic features

- Well-defined radiolucency with corticated borders
- From 25% to 40% involve an unerupted tooth

Treatment

There is no exact agreement that defines one treatment as a particular cure for the KCOT. Ideally, any treatment should remove the tumor as a whole, and then immediate subsequent treatment should remove any epithelial remnants and daughter cells.[15] When completed, the intraosseous framework should still be intact. Surgeons have tried to come to a consensus regarding the potential for recurrence of individual lesions. It seems that as the tumor size increases, so does the chance of recurrence; however, many investigators have found that tumor size does not correlate with recurrence.[15,16]

When managing pediatric patients, any treatment decision must take into account any unerupted teeth from the developing adult dentition. With recurrence rates as high as 25% to 60%, simple enucleation is not an acceptable mode of treatment.

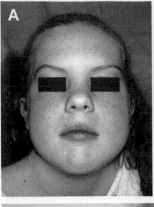
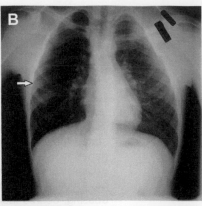
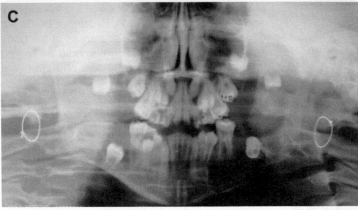

Fig. 7. (A) A 9-year-old girl showing classic features of BCNS: frontal bossing, broad nasal base, pseudohypertelorism, and mandibular prognathism. (B) The arrow points to bifid ribs. (C) Panorex shows KCOT lesions present in all 4 quadrants.

Marsupialization
- Tumors decrease in size, capsule may convert to orthokeratinized
- Marsupialization alone has around a 10% recurrence rate, which decreases when followed by a definitive procedure[13]
- Allows eruption and development of adult dentition

Enucleation and peripheral ostectomy
- Remove 1 to 2 mm of bone surrounding the visible margin
- Use methylene blue as a guide to remove adequate bone
- No adequate studies to define recurrence rate[13]

Carnoy solution
- Follows enucleation
- Leave in place for 5 minutes, irrigate with normal saline
- Damages inferior alveolar nerve if in contact for more than 2 minutes; protect with bone wax
- Studies show recurrence rate around 2.5%[13]

Cryotherapy
- Follows enucleation
- Liquid nitrogen penetrates 1.5 mm of bone

- If the inferior alveolar nerve is involved, nerve regeneration is excellent
- Recurrence rate around 10%[13]

Resection
- Recommended for large lesions with multiple perforations of the bony cortices
- Recurrence rate is 0%; however, overly aggressive for most lesions

Adenomatoid Odontogenic Tumor

Epidemiology
Although the literature contains numerous case reports, adenomatoid odontogenic tumor (AOT) is generally an uncommon tumor. Histologic examination of an AOT reveals a tumor of odontogenic epithelium with ductlike structures and potentially induced changes in the surrounding connective tissue.[17] Most of these lesions are associated with impacted teeth. It is seen often in the younger population, with 69% diagnosed in patients between the ages of 10 and 19 years. Of these, 53% are diagnosed in teenagers.[17]

Location
- More commonly associated with the maxilla than the mandible (2.1:1)

- Fifty-nine percent are associated with impacted canines (40% involve the maxillary canine)
- Unerupted first and second molars are rarely involved

Symptoms

- Asymptomatic
- Incidental radiographic finding on consultation for unerupted teeth

- May have gingival swelling, jaw enlargement, perforation of maxillary anterior bony cortices

Radiographic features

- Well-demarcated, unilocular radiolucency
- Seventy-one percent are pericoronal lesions (**Fig. 8**)
- Extracoronal lesions are located adjacent to roots, or may have no relationship to teeth

Treatment

AOTs are treated appropriately with enucleation and curettage. No recurrences have been reported in the literature, even with incomplete removal of the tumor.[18]

Calcifying Epithelial Odontogenic Tumor

Epidemiology

The calcifying epithelial odontogenic tumor (CEOT), also known as a Pindborg tumor, was first described in 1955 by the Dutch pathologist, Jens Jorgen Pindborg,[19] while he was investigating 3 benign, but locally invasive, intraosseous tumors. Before 1955, the tumor was reported under various names, because of the histologic variances. CEOT is the terminology used and adopted by the WHO.[20] Since the discovery of CEOT as a separate entity, a plethora of cases have been described in the literature.

Many histologic variants have been reported. Although benign, CEOT with findings of clear cells adjacent and joined to the epithelial cells with desmosomes may denote a more aggressive form of CEOT.[21,22] This finding may dictate a more aggressive form of treatment. In general, 94% of CEOTs are of the intraosseous type, and 60% of this type involves unerupted teeth. The remainder occur in an extraosseous location.

Philipsen and Reichart[23] reviewed 181 cases of CEOT from the literature. Their results revealed an age range of 8 to 92 years at the time of diagnosis, with a mean age of 36.9 years. Fewer than 15 cases were reported between the ages of 0 and 20 years.

Symptoms

- Intraosseous CEOT presents as painless, slow-growing mass
- Epistaxis, nasal stuffiness, and headaches are common complaints of patients with tumors presenting in the maxilla
- Extraosseous CEOT appears as a painless, firm gingival mass

Radiographic Features

- Unilocular/multilocular radiolucent lesion with radiopaque masses within the tumor

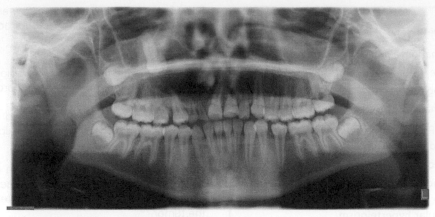

Fig. 8. Panorex shows an AOT in area #6 in a pediatric patient.

Treatment

Treatment of this tumor can be controversial because this tumor has the ability to recur if not adequately removed, which has led to comparisons with solid ameloblastoma, thus leading to recommendations for radical resection. Unlike the ameloblastoma, the CEOT has been shown to be an expansile lesion with no growth into the intertrabecular spaces.[24] Thick cortices of the mandible allow enucleation and curettage with peripheral ostectomy to be an acceptable treatment of a mandibular CEOT.

In the maxilla, the opposite is true: CEOTs do not remain well confined, and they tend to grow rapidly. The treatment of choice should be more aggressive, and surgical resection may be warranted.[23] Five-year follow-up is recommended after treatment.

Squamous Odontogenic Tumor

Epidemiology

This is an extremely rare tumor. According to Favia and colleagues,[25] only 36 cases have been described in the literature. These tumors generally occur in the third decade of life within the periodontium of permanent teeth, and only 1 case has been described associated with a deciduous tooth.[26] When these occur in the mandible, like most odontogenic tumors, there is a tendency for them to develop within the posterior regions (angle, ramus). When they occur in the maxilla, most squamous odontogenic tumors are located in the anterior maxilla.

Symptoms

- Swelling, pain
- Possible tooth mobility

Radiographic features

- Semicircular or triangular radiolucency

- Located in the alveolar process between the roots of corresponding teeth

Treatment

- Enucleation and curettage
- Must be histologically distinguished from primary intraosseous squamous cell carcinoma, which is very rare in the pediatric population

MIXED EPITHELIAL AND MESENCHYMAL ODONTOGENIC TUMORS

Mixed odontogenic tumors involve both the epithelial (enamel organ) and mesenchymal (dental papilla, dental follicle) components present during the process of odontogenesis. The most common clinical features include the absence of teeth, or positional anomalies of individual or groups of teeth, as well as swelling of the jaws.[27]

Odontoma

Epidemiology

Odontomas are considered to be the most common types of odontogenic tumors in the pediatric population. They tend to be discovered on routine radiographic examination during the first 2 decades of life. Rather than being described as true neoplasms, odontomas are considered hamartomatous developmental malformations of dental tissues. Odontomas consist primarily of enamel and dentin and are subdivided into 2 types: compound and complex. Compound odontomas are composed of organized collections of small tooth-like structures. Complex odontomas are composed of haphazard conglomerates of dental tissues (**Fig. 9**A). Compound odontomas most frequently occur in the anterior maxilla, whereas complex odontomas tend to develop in the posterior molar regions. They are most frequently

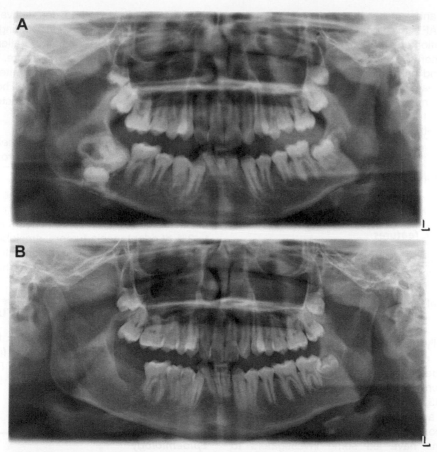

Fig. 9. (*A*) A 12-year-old boy with a complex odontoma in the right posterior mandible. (*B*) The same patient with the complex odontoma 3 months after enucleation and curettage showing complete resolution.

associated with disturbances in tooth eruption. In studies by Katz,[28] Tomizawa and colleagues,[29] and Kaugers and colleagues,[30] impacted teeth were associated with 41%, 47.6%, and 87% of odontomas, respectively. Compound odontomas are usually diagnosed radiographically, and are rarely confused with other lesions. However, complex odontomas can be confused with other highly calcified bone lesions, such as an osteoma.[4]

Symptoms

- Asymptomatic
- Delayed tooth eruption

Radiographic features

- Compound odontoma: calcified structures resembling teeth, usually surrounded by a narrow radiolucent zone associated with unerupted teeth
- Complex odontoma: dense, amorphous, irregularly shaped mass

Treatment

Treatment of odontomas consists of simple enucleation and curettage (**Fig. 9**B). Early detection of odontomas significantly increases the preservation of an associated impacted tooth, when present. An impacted tooth can be left to erupt; however, a secondary surgery may be necessary. Multiple studies have shown that spontaneous eruption of impacted teeth occurs in 32% to 45% of cases.[29,31] When a secondary procedure is necessary, it usually involves surgical exposure of the tooth crown, with or without the application of an orthodontic bracket and traction for forced eruption. In a study by Seo-Younf and Chang-Heon,[32] 100% of associated impacted teeth were able to be preserved in patients less than 9 years of age, whereas all impactions in patients more than the age of 30 years had to be removed.

Ameloblastic Fibroma

Epidemiology

Ameloblastic fibroma (AF) is considered a true neoplasm, in which both the odontogenic epithelial and mesenchymal elements are neoplastic. AF is most commonly seen in the pediatric population and represents only 2% of odontogenic tumors.[33] The mean age range is 6 to 12 years, and only a very few are seen after the age of 25 years.[34] AF most commonly occurs in the posterior mandible region. An incisional biopsy is warranted to rule out more aggressive lesions, which may influence the modality of treatment.

Symptoms

- Asymptomatic, slow-growing expansile lesion, typically discovered during routine radiographic examination

Radiographic features

- Unilocular or multilocular radiolucency with a well-defined sclerotic margin
- It may or may not be associated with the crown of an impacted tooth

Treatment

AF is usually treated appropriately with enucleation and curettage. Long-term follow-up is recommended because of the possibility of recurrence, which has been reported to range from 18.3% to 43.5%.[35] Most recurrences tend to be caused by an incomplete removal of the original lesion. Reports of transformation to ameloblastic fibrosarcoma have led some investigators to recommend a more aggressive approach with en bloc resection as the initial treatment of choice. Resection has also been recommended when the AF lesion is large and destructive in nature. Surgeons should be prudent in avoiding the developing tooth buds in pediatric patients during placement of reconstruction hardware. The reconstruction plate should be removed after 1 year to allow for growth, and any residual bony defect may be grafted and reconstructed, when indicated.[34]

Ameloblastic Fibro-odontoma, Ameloblastic Fibrodentinoma, Ameloblastic Fibrosarcoma

These mixed odontogenic tumors are considered variants of AF and are extremely rare. Although ameloblastic fibro-odontoma (AFO) and ameloblastic fibrodentinoma (AFD) account for only 1% to 3% of odontogenic tumors, ameloblastic fibrosarcoma (AFS) has been documented only 69 times in the literature as of 2012.[36] These tumors are summarized in **Table 1**.

MESENCHYMAL ODONTOGENIC TUMORS

Pediatric mesenchymal odontogenic tumors are rare and originate from the abnormal formation of the dental papilla and dental follicle. Each tumor is managed in an individual manner, because of the nature of the individual lesion.

Odontogenic Myxoma

Epidemiology

The odontogenic myxoma (OM) is an uncommon, benign, locally aggressive neoplasm arising from mesenchymal stroma, which accounts for 8.5%

Table 1
Less common types of mixed odontogenic tumors

	AFO	AFD	AFS
Tumor origin	Similar to AF. Also contains enamel and dentin	Similar to AF. Also contains dentin	Mesenchymal portion shows malignancy 1 in 3 develops de novo 2 in 3 are transformation from AF
Age	First and second decades	First and second decades	Third or fourth decades
Site	Posterior mandible (**Fig. 10**)	Posterior mandible	Posterior mandible
Symptoms	Disturbance in tooth eruption, jaw swelling	Disturbance in tooth eruption, jaw swelling	Pain, swelling, ulceration, parasthesia[37]
Treatment	E&C	E&C	Resection with margins 1.0–1.5 cm[34] Chemoradiation (controversial)
Recurrence	None expected	None expected	Up to 37%[38]

Abbreviation: E&C, enucleation and curettage.
Data from Refs.[34,37,38]

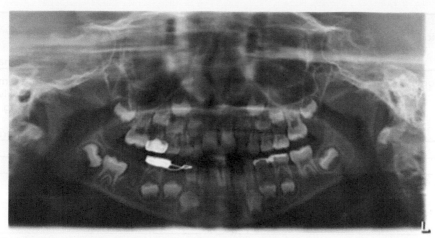

Fig. 10. An 8-year-old girl with an AFO in the right posterior mandible.

to 11.6% of pediatric odontogenic tumors.[39] Myxomas in general tend to occur in the myocardium. When they develop in the facial skeleton, the mandible is affected in two-thirds of cases, and the maxilla in one-third of cases.[40] The age distribution ranges from 5 to 65 years; however, most occur between the second and fourth decades of life.[34] On histology, OM presents as a nonencapsulated tumor consisting of an accumulation of mucoid ground substance with little collagen.[41]

In 2014 Kadlub and colleagues[42] also highlighted the occurrence of OM in infants (aged ≤2 years), suggesting a specific entity, infant OM. The major differences seen in infants include rapid development and a location limited to the maxilla.

Symptoms

- Slow, painless bony expansion with resultant facial deformity
- May be associated with an unerupted tooth

Radiographic features

- Multilocular radiolucency often described as honeycombed (or soap bubble)

Treatment

Treatment of this tumor is controversial. Typical management consists of surgical resection with 1.0-mm to 1.5-mm bony margins, and a margin of 1 uninvolved anatomic barrier is considered a curative surgery.[34] Recurrence rates have been reported to be up to 25%; however, this is with conservative treatment of enucleation and curettage.[40] Seeding of the tumor has been shown to locally invade the cancellous bone, which is why initial surgical resection is recommended. Some surgeons may be reluctant to perform a wide surgical excision in children for concern about facial disfigurement or interference with facial growth; however, secondary surgeries can have serious consequences because of the risk of seeding the tumor into unresectable anatomic spaces.[34,40]

Cementoblastoma

Epidemiology

Cementoblastoma is a rare, benign, odontogenic tumor that typically forms around the apical half of a vital tooth root. The neoplasm is often referred to as a true cementoma, and comprises less than 1% of all odontogenic tumors. Cementoblastoma almost always involves the permanent dentition; however, 5 cases affecting deciduous teeth have been recorded in the literature.[43] The age distribution ranges from the first to third decades of life.[34] Several case series have shown the mandibular first permanent molar to be involved more than 50% of the time.[43] On histology, the neoplasm is characterized by the formation of sheets of cementumlike tissue containing a large number of reversal lines and a lack of mineralization at the periphery of the mass or in the more active growth center.[44]

Symptoms

- Asymptomatic versus deep, dull pain
- Most commonly occurs in posterior mandible
- Hard expansion of the jaw is commonly seen
- Tooth is vital

Radiographic features

- Radiopaque mass fused to the apical half of the root, surrounded and limited peripherally by a radiolucent halo

Table 2
Classification of central and peripheral odontogenic fibroma

	Central Odontogenic Fibroma	Peripheral Odontogenic Fibroma
Epidemiology	• Very rare • Few reported cases in literature • 1 in 3 associated with unerupted tooth[4]	• Originates from periodontal membrane • Firm soft tissue mass on gingiva, covered by normal-appearing mucosa • Considered a hamartoma • 175 cases reported in the literature[4]
Age	All ages	Second to seventh decades
Site	Both jaws	Premolar-canine region[34]
Symptoms	• Painless expansion of jaw • May displace tooth roots	Painless mass on gingiva
Radiographic Features	• Unilocular/multilocular radiolucency with well-defined borders (**Fig. 11**)	NA
Treatment	E&C	Excision
Recurrence	None expected	None expected, if lesion completely excised

Abbreviation: NA, not available.
   Data from Neville B, Damm D, Allen C, et al. Oral and maxillofacial pathology. Philadelphia: WB Saunders; 1996; and Marx R, Stern D. Oral and maxillofacial pathology: a rationale for diagnosis and treatment. 2nd edition. Chicago: Quintessence; 2012.

Treatment

Cementoblastomas have an unlimited growth potential and require surgical removal along with the involved tooth. The growth rate is estimated to be 0.5 cm per year.[45] The tumor can usually be removed in 1 unit with the tooth attached to the lesion. The buccal cortex around the tumor may be absent or severely thinned, which may require a bone graft.[34] Recurrence is not expected, unless a portion of the tumor is left behind. Brannon and colleagues[45] reviewed a case series of 44 recurrent cementoblastomas and recommended a peripheral ostectomy, in addition to surgical removal, to reduce the chance of recurrence.

Central and Peripheral Odontogenic Fibroma

Central and peripheral odontogenic fibroma are summarized in **Table 2**.

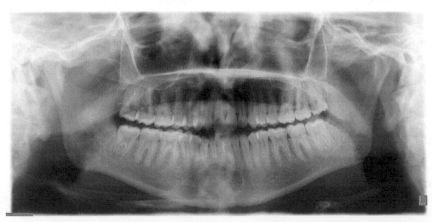

Fig. 11. Central odontogenic fibroma located in the anterior mandible with minor root displacement.

REFERENCES

1. Marx R. Jaw cysts, benign odontogenic tumors of the jaws, and fibro-osseous diseases. In: Bagheri SC, Bell RB, Khan HA, editors. Current therapy in oral and maxillofacial surgery. St Louis (MO): Elsevier Saunders; 2012. p. 399.

2. Sato M, Tanaka N, Sato T, et al. Oral and maxillofacial tumors in children: a review. Br J Oral Maxillofac Surg 1997;63:92–5.

3. Tanaka N, Murata A, Yamaguchi A, et al. Clinical features and management of oral and maxillofacial tumors in children. Oral Surg Oral Med Oral Pathol Oral Radiol Endod 1999;88:11–5.

4. Neville B, Damm D, Allen C, et al. Oral and maxillofacial pathology. Philadelphia: WB Saunders; 1996.

5. Bansal S, Desai RS, Shirstat P, et al. The occurrence and pattern of ameloblastoma in children and adolescents: an Indian institutional study of 41 years and review of the literature. Int J Oral Maxillofac Surg 2015;44(6):725–31.

6. Ackerman GL, Altini M, Shear M. The unicystic ameloblastoma: a clinicopathological study of 57 cases. J Oral Pathol 1988;17:541–6.

7. Ord RA, Blanchaert RH, Nikitakis NG, et al. Ameloblastoma in children. J Oral Maxillofac Surg 2002; 60:762–70.

8. Yazar S, Wei FC, Cheng MH, et al. Safety and reliability of microsurgical free tissue transfers in paediatric head and neck reconstruction: a report of 72 cases. J Plast Reconstr Surg 2008;61:767–71.

9. Jayaraj G, Sherlin HJ, Ramani P, et al. Metastasizing ameloblastoma: a perennial pathological enigma? Report of a case and review of literature. J Craniomaxillofac Surg 2014;42:772–9.

10. Bruce AB, Jackson T. Ameloblastic carcinoma: a report of an aggressive case and review of the literature. J Craniomaxillofac Surg 1991;19:267–71.

11. Sozzi D, Morganti V, Valente GM, et al. Ameloblastic carcinoma in a young patient. Oral Surg Oral Med Oral Pathol Oral Radiol 2014;117: e396–402.

12. Philipsen HP. Om keratocystedr (Kolesteratomer) and kaeberne. Tandlaegebladet 1956;60:963–71.

13. Pogrel MA. The keratocystic tumor. Oral Maxillofac Surg Clin North Am 2013;25:21–30.

14. Suzuki M, Nagao K, Hatsuse H, et al. Molecular odontogenic tumors developing in nevoid basal cell carcinoma syndrome. Oral Surg Oral Med Oral Pathol Oral Radiol 2013;116:348–53.

15. Kaczmarzyk T, Mojsa I, Stypulkowska J. A systematic review of the recurrence rate for keratocystic odontogenic tumor in relation to treatment modalities. Int J Oral Maxillofac Surg 2012;41:765–7.

16. Anand VK, Arrowood JP Jr, Krolls SO. Odontogenic keratocysts: a study of 50 patients. Laryngoscope 1995;105:6–14.

17. Philipsen HP, Reichart PA. Adenomatoid odontogenic tumor: facts and figures. Oral Oncol 1998; 35:125–31.

18. Rick GM. Adenomatoid odontogenic tumor. Oral Maxillofac Surg Clin North Am 2004;16:333–53.

19. Pindborg JJ. Calcifying epithelial odontogenic tumors. Acta Pathol Microbiol Scand Suppl 1955;111:71.

20. Pindborg JJ, Kramer IR. Histological typing of odontogenic tumors, jaw cysts, and allied lesions. Geneva (Switzerland): World Health Organization; 1971.

21. Waldron CA, Silverman H. Clear cell ameloblastoma: an odontogenic carcinoma. J Oral Maxillofac Surg 1985;43:701–17.

22. Hansen LS, Eversole LR, Green TL, et al. Clear cell odontogenic tumor: a new histological variant with aggressive potential. Head Neck Surg 1985; 8:115–23.

23. Philipsen HP, Reichart PA. Calcifying odontogenic tumor: biological profile based on 181 cases from the literature. Oral Oncol 2000;36:17–26.

24. Vap DR, Dahlin DC, Turlington EG. Pindborg tumor: the so-called calcifying epithelial odontogenic tumor. Cancer 1970;25:629–36.

25. Favia GF, Alberti DI, Scarano A, et al. Squamous odontogenic tumor: report of two cases. Oral Oncol 1997;33:451–3.

26. Philipsen HP, Reichart PA. Squamous odontogenic tumor (SOT): a benign neoplasm of the periodontium. A review of 36 reported cases. J Clin Periodontol 1996;23:922–6.

27. Gyulai-Gaal S, Takacs D, Szabo G, et al. Mixed odontogenic tumors in children and adolescents. J Craniofac Surg 2007;18(6):1338–42.

28. Katz RW. An analysis of compound and complex odontomas. J Dent Child 1989;56(6):445–9.

29. Tomizawa M, Otsuka Y, Noda T. Clinical observations of odontomas in Japanese children: 39 cases including one recurrent case. Int J Paediatr Dent 2005;15:37–43.

30. Kaugers GE, Miller ME, Abbey LM. Odontomas. Oral Surg 1989;67:172–6.

31. Morning P. Impacted teeth in relation to odontomas. Int J Oral Surg 1980;9:81–91.

32. Seo-Young AN, Chang-Heon AN. Karp-Shik Choi. Odontoma: a retrospective study of 73 cases. Imaging Sci Dent 2012;42:277–81.

33. Blankestijn J, Panders AK, Wymenga JP. Ameloblastic fibroma of the mandible. Br J Oral Maxillofac Surg 1986;24:417.

34. Marx R, Stern D. Oral and maxillofacial pathology: a rationale for diagnosis and treatment. 2nd edition. Chicago: Quintessence; 2012.

35. Pereira K, Bennett K, Elkins T, et al. Ameloblastic fibroma of the maxillary sinus. Int J Pediatr Otorhinolaryngol 2004;68:1473–7.

36. Lai J, Blanas N, Higgins K, et al. Ameloblastic fibrosarcoma: report of a case, study of

immunophenotype, and comprehensive review of the literature. J Oral Maxillofac Surg 2012;70: 2007–12.

37. Noordhoek R, Pizer M, Laskin D. Ameloblastic fibrosarcoma of the mandible: treatment, long-term follow up, and subsequent reconstruction of a case. J Oral Maxillofac Surg 2012;70:2930–5.

38. Bregni RC, Taylor AM, García AM. Ameloblastic fibrosarcoma of the mandible: report of two cases and review of the literature. J Oral Pathol Med 2001;30:316.

39. Mortellaro C, Berrone M, Turatti G, et al. Odontogenic tumors in childhood: a retrospective study of 86 treated cases. Importance of a correct histopathologic diagnosis. J Craniofac Surg 2008;19(4): 1173e–6e.

40. King T, Lewis J, Orvidas L, et al. Pediatric maxillary odontogenic myxoma: a report of 2 cases and review of management. J Oral Maxillofac Surg 2008; 66:1057–62.

41. Simon E, Merkx AW, Vuhahula E, et al. Odontogenic myxoma: a clinicopathological study of 33 cases. In J Oral Maxillofac Surg 2004;33:333–7.

42. Kadlub N, Mbou VB, Leboulanger N, et al. Infan odontogenic myxoma: a specific entity J Craniomaxillofac Surg 2014;42:2082–6.

43. Schafer T, Singh B, Myers D. Cementoblastoma associated with a primary tooth: a rare pediatric lesion. Pediatr Dent 2001;23:351–3.

44. Kramer IR, Pindborg JJ, Shear M. Histologica typing of odontogenic tumors. In: World Health Organization International histological classification of tumors. 2nd edition. New York: Springer-Verlag Berlin Heidelberg 1992. p. 23.

45. Brannon R, Fowler C, Carpenter W, et al. Cementoblastoma: an innocuous neoplasm? A clinicopathologic study of 44 cases and review of the literature with special emphasis on recurrence. Oral Pathol Oral Radiol Endod 2002;93 311–20.

Nonodontogenic Tumors of the Jaws

Donita Dyalram, DDS, MD, FACS*, Nawaf Aslam-Pervez, DDS, MD,
Joshua E. Lubek, DDS, MD, FACS

KEYWORDS

- Fibro-osseous lesions • Giant cell lesions • Desmoplastic lesions • Nonodontogenic tumors

KEY POINTS

- Nonodontogenic tumors of the jaws are common in the pediatric population; these tumors include giant cell lesions, fibro-osseous lesions, and desmoplastic fibroma.
- Giant cell lesions of the maxillofacial skeleton range clinically from slowly growing, asymptomatic radiolucency discovered on routine radiographs to rapidly expanding, aggressive tumors characterized by pain, root resorption, and a high recurrence rate.
- Fibro-osseous lesions represent a group of benign conditions that are characterized by replacement of normal bone with fibrous connective tissue that gradually undergoes mineralization.
- Desmoplastic fibroma is recognized as a benign bony neoplasm and as the intraosseous counterpart of soft tissue fibromatosis.

GIANT CELL LESIONS

Introduction

Giant cell lesions of the maxillofacial skeleton range clinically from slowly growing, asymptomatic radiolucency discovered on routine radiographs to rapidly expanding, aggressive tumors characterized by pain, root resorption, and a high recurrence rate. They are generally considered to be nonneoplastic, although some lesions tend to behave aggressively like a neoplasm. Names such as central giant cell granuloma, giant cell lesion, giant cell tumor, or giant cell reparative granuloma have added to the complexity and confusion of this lesion. The reparative term has been rejected in recent times because the lesions are typically destructive and aggressive, never reparative. The term granuloma is also a misnomer; however, the central giant cell granuloma has now become synonymous with a lesion in the maxillofacial skeleton.

Nature of the Problem

When considering these types of lesions it is important to keep in mind (1) brown tumor of hyperparathyroidism, (2) central giant cell granuloma, (3) giant cell tumor, and (4) cherubism, which are distinct clinical entities that should be part of every differential diagnosis. Giant cell lesions are distinct biologically from the aggressive and frequently malignant giant cell lesions of the extremities, which are also called giant cell tumors.

Central giant cell granuloma (CGCG) was first described by Jaffe[1] in 1953 as a reparative granuloma to convey that it was not a neoplasm.[2] The central giant cell lesion is a benign localized proliferation that is osteolytic and sometimes aggressive, consisting of fibrous tissue containing multinucleated giant cells, hemorrhagic areas, and deposits of hemosiderin, and occasionally involving a bone reaction.[2]

Clinical Findings

These lesions occur in all ages; however, they are seen predominantly in children and young adults and are usually diagnosed before 30 years of age.[3] Female patients are affected more often than male patients, and some studies have shown a rate of

Department of Oral Maxillofacial Surgery, University of Maryland Dental School, 650 West Baltimore Street, Room 1218, Baltimore, MD 21201, USA
* Corresponding author.
E-mail address: ddyalram@umaryland.edu

Oral Maxillofacial Surg Clin N Am 28 (2016) 59–65
http://dx.doi.org/10.1016/j.coms.2015.08.002
1042-3699/16/$ – see front matter © 2016 Elsevier Inc. All rights reserved.

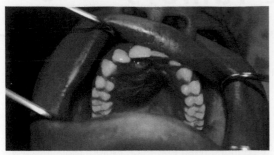

Fig. 1. Intraoral view of a CGCG of the right maxilla in a 14-year-old child. Note the expansion of the palate, and the bluish hue of the overlying intact mucosa.

about 60% in women. The mandible is affected more often than the maxilla. The premolar and molar regions of the mandible are more affected than the ascending ramus region, and, rarely, there is involvement of the mandibular condyle or the maxillary sinus. In most cases it presents as an asymptomatic lesion detected on routine radiographic examination; however, pain, paresthesia, perforation of cortical bone, mobility, and loss of teeth are reported in aggressive lesions (**Figs. 1** and **2**).

Demographics:

- Predilection for women
- Occurrence in the first 3 decades of life
- Mandible more than maxilla, most often anterior to the first molar
- Most often a solitary lesion

Physical examination:

- Asymptomatic, but can be associated with discomfort, pain, paresthesia
- Teeth can be displaced or nonvital
- Maxillary lesions may present as nasal obstruction or epistaxis
- May present as a bulge of the alveolar ridge

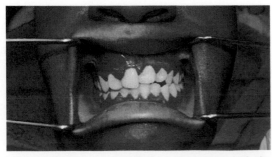

Fig. 2. Alternate view of the same CGCG of the maxilla in **Fig. 1**, showing the expansion of the alveolar ridge and displaced dentition.

Imaging

Radiographically, these lesions are usually mixed radiolucent/radio-opaque and multilocular. Other findings have been described, such as loss of lamina dura, root resorption, and displacement of teeth, and cases with localization in the region mimicking periapical cysts or periapical granulomas have been reported. They typically appear as an expansile radiolucency with scalloped margins containing numerous thin septa of wispy bone and osteoid (**Fig. 3**).

Characteristic findings on radiographs:

- Loss of lamina dura
- Resorption of teeth in aggressive lesions
- Smooth or scalloped margins
- Ill defined or corticated
- Can cross the midline
- Contains numerous thin septa of wispy bone and osteoid

Pathology

A giant cell lesion is a localized tumor of multinucleated giant cells that represent osteoclasts in a matrix of spindle-shaped mesenchymal cells.[4]

Histopathology[5]:

- Lobulated bluish mass of proliferating vascular connective tissue
- Osteoclastlike giant cells
- Hemosiderin deposition
- Spindle-shaped fibroblastic or myofibroblastic cells in a fibrous or fibromyxoid vascularized tissue

Diagnostic Dilemma

Several other lesions can resemble a giant cell lesion microscopically and must be considered in the differential diagnosis (**Box 1**).

Brown tumor of hyperparathyroidism

It is histologically indistinguishable from CGCG. In the pediatric population this is associated with chronic renal failure and secondary hyperparathyroidism. Primary hyperparathyroidism is rare in children. This lesion is a result of bone resorption in a setting of increased parathyroid hormone level. To help to differentiate this tumor, serum calcium and alkaline phosphate levels are increased and serum phosphate levels are low. Chronically increased serum creatinine and blood urea nitrogen levels are also seen in patients with chronic renal disease.

Cherubism

This is indistinguishable from CGCG; however, lesions are symmetric and occur near the angles of the mandible. They do not affect the condyle or the body of the mandible. In the maxilla the

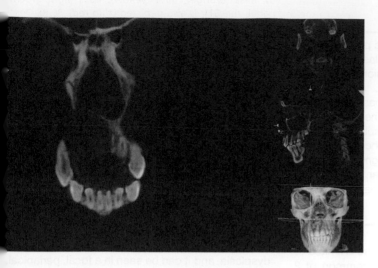

Fig. 3. Cone beam computed tomography (CT) of the same patient in **Figs. 1** and **2**, showing an expansile mass in the left anterior maxilla. Notice the well defined borders of the lesion crossing the midline as well as the thinning of the cortical bone.

tuberosities are affected and sometimes the anterior portion of the orbits. It is an autosomal dominant familial disease and has been mapped to chromosome 4p16.3, which codes for a c-Abl binding protein.[6] It is seen in early childhood, as early as 14 months. These lesions regress as the patient ages and bone growth ceases.

Aneurysmal bone cysts

These lesions are seen mostly in patients younger than 30 years, with peak occurrence in the second decade. These lesions on histologic examination contain giant cells as well as reactive bone. It is unlikely that they are result of trauma and some of them are considered to be neoplastic. They are localized mostly to the posterior mandible and radiographically appear unilocular or multilocular, predominantly radiolucent. The involvement of soft tissue increases the chances of recurrences.

Fibrous dysplasia

On histologic examination they have limited foci of giant cells. They can also appear similarly on radiographs during the early stages (discussed in depth later).

Treatment

Clinicians must take into account the behavior, clinical components, and biological components of the giant cell lesions when determining how to manage them. For all intents and purposes, clinicians attempt to identify giant cell lesions as either aggressive or nonaggressive. Nonaggressive giant cell lesions predictably respond to enucleation and curettage. Adjuvant therapies such as steroids or calcitonin are rarely used because patients with nonaggressive lesions typically respond to curettage and enucleation alone. Recurrence for these lesions is low. Aggressive giant cell lesions clinically present as rapidly expanding masses in younger patients. These giant cell lesions should be resected with a 1.0-cm histologically clear margin. Postoperative adjuncts such as bisphosphonates, intralesional steroid injection, calcitonin therapy, or systemic interferon alfa therapy have all been reported with various levels of success. Brown tumor of hyperparathyroidism can be treated by curettage but usually regresses once the endocrine abnormality has resolved.

FIBRO-OSSEOUS LESION
Introduction

Fibro-osseous lesions (FOLs) of the craniofacial complex represent a group of benign conditions that are characterized by replacement of normal bone with fibrous connective tissue that gradually undergoes mineralization. The name given to this group presents a process rather than a diagnosis.

Box 1
Nonodontogenic tumors of the jaw

Giant cell lesions

- CGCG
- Brown tumor of hyperparathyroidism
- Cherubism

Fibro-osseous lesions

- Fibrous dysplasia
- Ossifying fibroma
- Osseous dysplasia

Desmoplastic fibroma

Nature of the Problem

The subtypes of these benign FOLs present similar microscopic features, but clinical classification has represented a challenge. These lesions are fibrous dysplasia (FD), ossifying fibroma, and osseous dysplasia.[7] Each of these subtypes has different clinical and radiological presentations. They show a wide range of biological behavior from dysplasia to benign neoplasia with occasional recurrence. Radiologic examination is central to their diagnosis because histopathology for all FOLs is similar. Furthermore, once diagnosed the management of each is different.

Fibrous Dysplasia

Monostotic fibrous dysplasia

As described by its name, this disease is limited to 1 bone. This disease is the most common of 2 types with an incidence of 80% of reported cases. The jaws are the most commonly involved bone, in particular the maxilla. They are associated with the GNAS1, which can occur anytime during pregnancy, childhood, or adulthood.

Polyostotic fibrous dysplasia

FD is considered polyostotic once 2 or more bones are involved. It can be considering syndromic if other abnormalities are found:

1. Jaffe-Lichtenstein syndrome
   - Polyostotic FD
   - Café au lait spots
2. McCune-Albright syndrome
   - Polyostotic FD
   - Café au lait spots
   - Multiple endocrinopathies: sexual precocity, pituitary adenoma, and hyperthyroidism
3. Mazabraud syndrome
   - Polyostotic FD
   - Intramuscular myxomas

These children typically have a facial asymmetry. In the long bone counterpart, they are plagued with pathologic fractures with ensuing pain and leg length discrepancy. Renal phosphate wasting is typically seen in these patients. This condition is caused by the release of fibroblast growth factor 23 (FGF23), which is produced and released by affected bone. The café au lait pigmentation is irregular (looking like the coast of Maine) compared with those of neurofibromatosis, which are regular (like the coast of California).

Ossifying Fibroma

Of all the FOLs discussed in this article, this one represents a true neoplasm. A discussion of this lesion is not complete without noting its pediatric counterpart. It is generally accepted that there are 2 forms

based on histology and clinical behavior. They are the trabecular ossifying fibroma (TOF) and psammomatoid ossifying fibroma (POF). They were first distinguished by El-Mofty[8] as 2 entities based on histology and age. TOF occurs mostly in children 8 to 12 years old and POF in those 16 to 33 years old. Most of the reported cases of POF occur in the orbit, paranasal sinus, and calvaria, with only 25% in the maxilla and mandible. TOF overwhelming occurs in the jaws, in particular the maxilla. Radiographically these lesions are indistinguishable.

Osseous Dysplasia

These lesions are rarely seen in the pediatric population but are categorized with the FOLs. Other names for this disease include cemento-osseous dysplasia, and it can be seen in a focal, periapical, or florid pattern, hence the names: focal cemento-osseous dysplasia, periapical cemento-osseous dysplasia or cementoma, or cemental dysplasia; and florid cemento-osseous dysplasia.

Clinical Findings

These lesions are benign and noninheritable. They are typically seen in the second and third decades, with the pediatric variant seen much earlier. There is an equal male/female predilection in FD, whereas ossifying fibroma tends to occur mostly in female patients and in the mandibles. Small lesions are discovered as incident findings on radiographs. Larger lesions presents as painless swelling of the involved bone. There is usually a resultant facial asymmetry, which is striking in some cases.

Imaging

The radiographic appearances of these lesions have been key to helping with the diagnosis and ultimately the management. They typically have varying degrees of radio-opacity based on their maturity (**Figs. 4–6**).

Characteristic findings on radiographs:

FD:
- Ground-glass appearance
- Expansion of buccal and lingual cortices
- Displacement of the inferior alveolar canal
- Ill-defined lamina dura
- Not well demarcated from adjacent tissue
- Radiolucent or mixed

Ossifying fibroma
- Well demarcated
- Unilocular with sclerotic border
- Can be radiolucent or radio-opaque
- Root resorption or divergence possible

Osseous dysplasia
- Mixed radiolucent/radiopaque

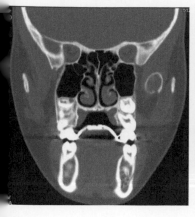
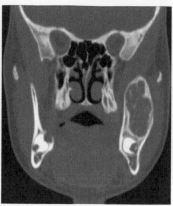

Fig. 4. CT scan, coronal view, of a 13-year-old girl of a mixed radiolucent/radio-opaque lesion in the left posterior mandible, extending from the angle of the mandible to the coronoid process but sparing the condyle. The time difference between the images is 6 months. Note the well-defined borders of the lesion. This patient underwent a resection of the lesion, which proved to be an ossifying fibroma.

- Well defined with irregular borders
- Usually associated with dentition

Pathology

On histology these two lesions are similar in appearance, with irregular trabeculae of woven bone in a fibrous stroma. These trabeculae are not connected, are curvilinear, and appear haphazard, in contrast with the ossifying fibroma. In FD, this diseased bone is fused to normal bone.

In the juvenile ossifying fibroma, the stromal background is similar in that it is of fibrous connective tissue and it is the mineralized component that identifies the 2 entities. For TOF, the osteoids are irregular, cellular, and lined by osteoblasts. The POF is noted for having concentric ossicles of varying sizes with a basophilic center and eosinophilic rim.

Treatment

Management of FOLs depends on their diagnosis. The histopathology is often limited in aiding the diagnostic dilemma. It is critical to put the entire clinical picture together to arrive at the diagnosis and hence render the appropriate treatment.

For FD, this can be particularly challenging in cases that are polyostotic and involve the craniofacial bones. With skeletal maturity the growth of these bones tends to stabilize. The cosmetic deformity, ensuing psychological issues, and function problems are what drive the surgical intervention. Despite recontouring, there are reported cases of 25% to 50% regrowth of the bone, especially when this is done at a young age. For the polyostotic variant, treatment with intravenous pamidronate and oral alendronate have shown success, especially in pain relief and skeletal strength. Clinicians must keep in mind the risk of transformation to osteosarcoma if it is treated with radiotherapy.

The treatment of ossifying fibroma involves enucleation of the tumor. If there is considerable bony destruction, resection and bone grafting are warranted. The prognosis is good and the rate of recurrence is slow. There is no reported case of malignant transformation of ossifying fibroma.

DESMOPLASTIC FIBROMA

Desmoplastic fibroma is recognized as a benign bony neoplasm and as the intraosseous

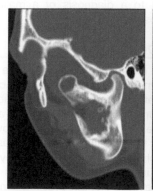
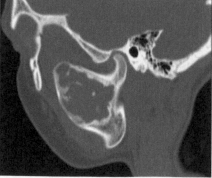

Fig. 5. CT scan of the same patient from **Fig. 4**, sagittal cut, showing destruction of the coronoid process.

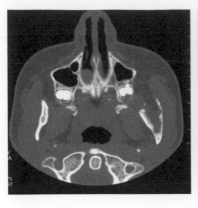

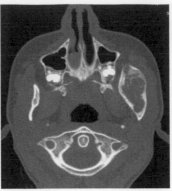

Fig. 6. Axial view of the ossifying fibroma showing expansion of the coronoid process and the typical mixed radiolucent/radio-opaque pattern.

counterpart of soft tissue fibromatosis. It has a locally aggressive behavior and a high recurrence rate. It is rare, with an incidence of less than 1% of all bone tumors.[9] This fibroma represents the osseous manifestation of aggressive fibromatosis that was first reported by Jaffe[10] in 1958.[10,11]

Clinical Findings

The desmoplastic fibroma is typically seen in the younger population with an average age around 16 years. There is no sex predilection. These lesions are commonly seen in the mandible (22%), femur (15%), pelvic bones (13%), radius (12%), and tibia (9%),[9] with the ascending ramus being the most common of the gnathic sites. Typically they present as a painless swelling with symptoms presenting as the tumor invades adjacent structures[12] (**Fig. 7**).

Physical examination:

- Asymptomatic: 65%
- Pain: 15%

- Trismus with or without malocclusion: 11%
- Tooth mobility: 7%
- Dysesthesia: 2.65%
- Proptosis, elevated earlobe, infection: 2.6%

Imaging

They appear as a multilocular, occasionally unilocular, radiolucent area. There is expansion and thinning of the cortices and the borders of the lesions can be well or ill defined. If left long enough, perforation of the cortices will occur (**Fig. 8**). The adjacent teeth can show displacement and root resorption. This condition often mimics other jaw disorders like ameloblastoma, odontogenic myxoma, aneurysmal bone cyst, and central hemangioma.

Pathology

This tumor consists of abundant collagen fibers and fibroblasts. The degree of cellularity may vary in different regions of these lesions. At the periphery of the lesion, reactive bone can be seen and this can be confused with an FOL if biopsy size is inadequate. This tumor lacks abundant cellular pleomorphism, hyperchromatism, and mitotic figures. An increase in atypical cells can lead to a diagnosis of a malignancy, such as fibrosarcoma.

Diagnostic Dilemma

The diagnostic dilemma in the management of desmoplastic fibroma lies in the challenge in differentiating it from a low-grade fibrosarcoma. This lesion has a similar clinical and radiographic appearance. This lesion is a slow-growing malignant tumor of fibroblasts, often asymptomatic until reaching a significant size. They most commonly occur in the paranasal sinuses and nose, which is the reason for late presentation or nasal obstructive symptoms. Like desmoplastic fibroma, they

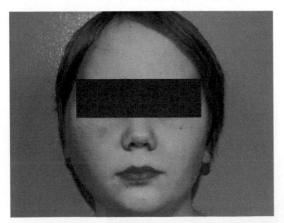

Fig. 7. A child showing an expansile mass in the right midface. Note the loss of the nasolabial groove, and fullness over the malar region.

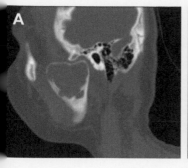 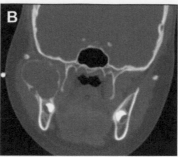

Fig. 8. CT scan. Sagittal (*A*) and coronal (*B*) views of a desmoplastic fibroma of the right posterior mandible. Note the erosion and perforation of the cortical plates of this radiolucent lesion.

are commonly seen in the pediatric population. On histology, they have spindle-shaped cells that form a herring-bone pattern, whereas desmoplastic fibroma favors a single-cell pattern. There is increase in mitotic figures, pleomorphism, and decreased collagenous background. In the cases in which the desmoplastic fibroma extends into the soft tissue, the clinical picture can be confused. Treatment of fibrosarcoma is resection with wide margin, with 5-year survival ranging from 40% to 50%.

Treatment

This is a benign, aggressive lesion that is locally destructive and easily extends into soft tissue. Therefore treatment of desmoplastic fibroma is resection of the lesion with margins. Some clinicians have argued that treatment of desmoplastic fibroma, confined within the bone, with curettage has a 70% recurrence rate, whereas resection with margins has shown recurrence rates around 20%.[12] Radiotherapy and chemotherapy have also been proposed, with limited success and risk for malignant transformation.[13] For this reason, these patients need to be followed for several years.

ACKNOWLEDGMENTS

The authors thank Dr John Caccamese for his assistance with providing the photographs and computed tomography scans for this article.

REFERENCES

1. Jaffe HL. Giant-cell reparative granuloma, traumatic bone cyst and fibrous dysplasia of the jaw bones. Oral Surg Oral Med Oral Pathol 1953;6:159–75.

2. Kadluba N. Specificity of paediatric jawbone lesions: tumours and pseudotumours. J Craniomaxillofac Surg 2014;42(2):125–31.

3. De Lange J. Incidence and disease-free survival after surgical therapy of central giant cell granulomas of the jaws in the Netherlands: 1990-1995. Head Neck 2004;26:792–5.

4. Barnes L, Eveson JW, Reichart P, editors. WHO classification of tumors. Lyon (France): ARC Press; 2005.

5. Chuong R. Central giant cell lesions of the jaws: a clinicopathologic study. J Oral Maxillofac Surg 1986;44:157–63.

6. Mangion J. The gene for cherubism maps to chromosome 4p16.3. Am J Hum Genet 1999;65:151–7.

7. MacDonald-Jankowski DS. Fibro-osseous lesions of the face and jaws. Clin Radiol 2004;59(1):11–25.

8. El-Mofty S. Psammomatoid and trabecular juvenile ossifying fibroma of the craniofacial skeleton: two distinct clinicopathologic entities. Oral Surg Oral Med Oral Pathol Oral Radiol Endod 2002;93(3): 296–304.

9. Bohm P. Desmoplastic fibroma of the bone: a report of two patients, review of the literature and therapeutic implications. Cancer 1996;78:1011–23.

10. Jaffe HL. Tumors and timorous conditions of the bones and joints. Philadelphia: Lea and Febiger; 1958. p. 298.

11. Said-Al-Naief N. Desmoplastic fibroma of the jaw: a case report and review of the literature. Oral Surg Oral Med Oral Pathol Oral Radiol Endod 2006;101: 82–94.

12. Iwai S. Desmoplastic fibroma of the mandible mimicking osteogenic sarcoma: report of a case. J Oral Maxillofac Surg 1996;54:1370–3.

13. Ayala AG. Desmoid fibromatosis: clinicopathologic study of 25 children. Semin Diagn Pathol 1886;3: 138–50.

Benign Pediatric Salivary Gland Lesions

Eric R. Carlson, DMD, MD[a],*, Robert A. Ord, DDS, MD, FRCS, MS, MBA[b]

KEYWORDS

- Mucocele • Ranula • Sialolithiasis • Sialadenitis • Pleomorphic adenoma • Hemangioma

KEY POINTS

- Salivary gland lesions are uncommonly observed in the pediatric population, and benign salivary gland lesions are more common than malignant salivary gland lesions in children.
- The mucocele is the most common salivary gland lesion encountered in pediatric patients.
- Mumps has historically been the most common form of sialadenitis diagnosed in children internationally.
- Chronic recurrent parotitis is the second most common form of sialadenitis in children.
- The pleomorphic adenoma is the most common pediatric salivary gland tumor and the most common benign tumor in children. Together with the hemangioma, these benign tumors account for nearly 90% of all benign salivary gland tumors in children.

INTRODUCTION

Diseases of the salivary glands are uncommonly observed in pediatric patients. In 1972 the Armed Forces Institute of Pathology (AFIP) identified 430 salivary gland lesions in children younger than the age of 15 years in their study of 9983 salivary gland lesions, accounting for only 4.3% of the total.[1] This study identified 262 nonneoplastic lesions (61%), among which there were 185 mucoceles (71%) and 67 inflammatory lesions (26%). Of the 430 salivary gland lesions, 168 salivary gland tumors (39%) were noted, of which 114 tumors were benign (68%) and 54 tumors were malignant (32%). Sixty of the 114 (53%) benign tumors in this series were epithelial in nature and 39 (34%) represented vascular proliferations. Pleomorphic adenoma was the most common benign tumor in this series and the most common malignant tumor was mucoepidermoid carcinoma. In 1991, Ellis and colleagues[2] reviewed benign and malignant salivary gland tumors in patients less than the age of 17 years and compared these tumors and their frequency with patients of all ages. These pediatric patients accounted for only 4.5% of all patients with salivary gland lesions in their series. A total of 494 salivary gland tumors were reviewed, of which 271 (55%) were benign tumors. These tumors included 210 (78%) benign epithelial tumors and 61 (22%) benign mesenchymal tumors. Pleomorphic adenomas accounted for 193 cases (39%) occurring in this age group and 71% of all benign tumors in this series. The pleomorphic adenomas represented only 3.9% of these tumors occurring in all age groups, owing to the greater percentage of other benign tumors occurring in patients younger than 17 years of age. Two-hundred and twenty-three tumors were malignant (45%), with 212 (95%) being malignant epithelial tumors and 11 (5%) being malignant mesenchymal

[a] Department of Oral and Maxillofacial Surgery, University of Tennessee Medical Center, 1930 Alcoa Highway, Suite 335, Knoxville, TN 37920, USA; [b] Department of Oral and Maxillofacial Surgery, Baltimore College of Dental Surgery, University of Maryland and the Greenbaum Cancer Institute, Suite 1402, 650 W Baltimore Street, Suite 1218, Baltimore, MD 21201, USA
* Corresponding author. Department of Oral and Maxillofacial Surgery, University of Tennessee Medical Center, Suite 335, 1930 Alcoa Highway, Knoxville, TN 37920.
E-mail address: ecarlson@mc.utmck.edu

Oral Maxillofacial Surg Clin N Am 28 (2016) 67–81
http://dx.doi.org/10.1016/j.coms.2015.07.004
1042-3699/16/$ – see front matter © 2016 Elsevier Inc. All rights reserved.

tumors. Mucoepidermoid carcinoma accounted for 123 cases (25%) occurring in this age group and 55% of all malignant tumors in this series. Similarly, the mucoepidermoid carcinomas represented only 7.7% of these tumors occurring in all age groups owing to the greater percentage of other malignant tumors occurring in patients younger than 17 years of age.

Craver and Carr[3] reviewed 213 pediatric salivary gland lesions over a 17-year period and identified 173 nonneoplastic lesions (81%), of which there were 137 mucoceles (64% of total in series) and 26 inflammatory lesions (12% of total in series). There were 40 neoplasms, of which 36 (90%) were benign and 4 (10%) were malignant. The most common benign neoplasm was pleomorphic adenoma, accounting for 17 of the 36 cases (47%), followed by 12 cases of lymphangioma (33%). Of the 17 cases of pleomorphic adenoma, 11 were located in the parotid gland and 3 cases each were located in the submandibular gland and minor salivary glands.

In the African pediatric population, salivary gland neoplasms constitute 10% of all pediatric neoplasms. Most are reported to be benign, with the most common benign neoplasm being pleomorphic adenoma. Mumps has been reported as the most common inflammatory salivary gland lesion in Africa, but in the developed world only sporadic cases of mumps are now reported.[4]

In their series of 2135 patients with tumors of the major salivary glands from 1930 to 1964, Castro and colleagues[5] identified 38 patients (1.7%) 16 years of age and younger who were observed to have epithelial tumors. Thirty-three (87%) of the tumors were located in the parotid gland and 5 tumors (13%) were located in the submandibular gland. The most common benign tumor was pleomorphic adenoma and the most common malignant tumor was mucoepidermoid carcinoma. Lack and Upton[6] reported 80 salivary gland tumors in patients 18 years of age or younger during a 58-year period from 1928 to 1986. Twenty-five (31%) epithelial tumors were diagnosed and 55 (69%) nonepithelial tumors were diagnosed. Capillary hemangioma was the most common tumor diagnosed in this series, accounting for 27 (34%) of the 80 cases, followed by 19 cases of lymphangioma (24%), 10 cases (12.5%) of pleomorphic adenoma, and 6 cases (7.5%) of mucoepidermoid carcinoma.

NONNEOPLASTIC SALIVARY GLAND LESIONS

Nonneoplastic salivary gland lesions in children are associated with a wide spectrum of diagnoses and causes (**Box 1**). Congenital abnormalities, acute and chronic suppurative infections and

---

Box 1
Inflammatory and infectious diseases of the salivary glands in children

Viral infections

Paramyxovirus (mumps)

Coxsackie A and B

Echovirus

Influenza A

Cytomegalovirus

Epstein-Barr virus

Human immunodeficiency virus

Bacterial infections

Acute pyogenic infection

Recurrent parotitis

Intraparotid lymphadenopathy

Mycobacterium tuberculosis

Nontuberculous mycobacteria

Cat-scratch disease (*Bartonella henselae*)

Actinomycosis

Noninfectious disorders

Sarcoidosis

Sjögren syndrome

Pseudolymphomas

---

other inflammatory disorders, obstruction, neoplastic disease, and degenerative disorders should be considered as part of a differential diagnosis for a child with salivary gland swelling (**Fig. 1**). These nonneoplastic pathologic entities are less common in pediatric patients than in adults.[7] Inflammatory disorders of the salivary glands in children may be infectious or noninfectious. Infectious disorders may involve the parenchyma of the salivary gland as a sialadenitis, or the intrasalivary gland lymph nodes, as occurs in mycobacterium tuberculosis or with nontuberculous mycobacteria. Infectious disorders more commonly involve a single gland, as occurs in an acute bacterial parotitis, or a pair of major glands, as most commonly occurs in viral parotitis, such as that caused by paramyxovirus. Noninfectious inflammatory disease tends to involve multiple salivary glands, as occurs in Sjögren syndrome and sarcoidosis as a pansialadenitis.

Mucus Escape Reaction

The mucocele and ranula, collectively referred to as the mucus escape reaction, are most commonly diagnosed in the first and second

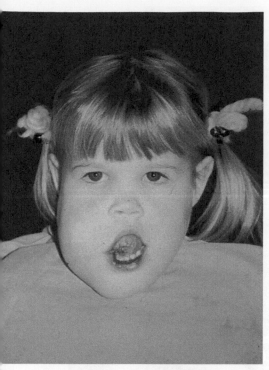

Fig. 1. A 4-year-old girl with a lymphangioma of the right parotid gland with extension into the right cheek and the tongue.

decades of life. Hayashida and colleagues[8] studied 173 cases of mucocele and found that 132 cases (76%) occurred in the first or second decades of life, with 49% of the mucoceles occurring in the second decade of life. Bhargava and colleagues[9] presented a case of a mucocele of the lower lip in an 11-month-old patient. Syebele and Butow[10] reviewed 50 cases of mucoceles and noted that 62% were diagnosed in the first 2 decades of life. Forty-eight of 50 patients were consented for human immunodeficiency virus (HIV) infection and 33 patients (68%) were HIV positive, 10 of whom were younger than 10 years of age. The investigators pointed out that mucoceles and ranulas might be considered, in the context of HIV-related salivary gland disease, as a group of lesions most commonly associated with HIV infection. They recommended consideration for HIV testing for all patients with oral mucoceles and ranulas. Because the number of patients studied in their series was low, additional information regarding the incidence of mucoceles and ranulas in patients infected with HIV seems warranted before recommending routine HIV testing of all patients with these benign salivary gland lesions.

In terms of treatment of the ranula, some investigators have recommended a 5-month to 6-month observation period in pediatric patients, after which time these patients should undergo surgical intervention if resolution has not occurred.[11,12] Seo and colleagues[13] reviewed 17 pediatric patients with symptomatic ranulas that exceeded 2 cm in diameter who underwent surgical excision of the ranula and offending sublingual gland. All patients had been observed for 3 to 14 months before being offered surgical intervention, and none of the cases underwent spontaneous resolution. In 2 cases the ranula increased in size. The investigators concluded that a lengthy presurgical observation period is not necessary in terms of surgical decision making for pediatric patients with ranulas. The low morbidity of sublingual gland excision as well as the lack of spontaneous resolution of the ranula supports surgical intervention, including sublingual gland excision, as its early and first-line therapy (**Fig. 2**).

Bacterial Sialadenitis

Bacterial sialadenitis is a rare disease in children. It most frequently involves the parotid gland. Newborn children, those with preexisting immunodeficiency or those receiving chemotherapy, and children with severe dental and gingival infections are particularly at risk for the development of bacterial sialadenitis. Physical examination reveals pain and swelling in the affected salivary gland. In their retrospective review of 118 patients aged 18 years and younger with parotid swellings, Orvidas and colleagues[14] reported 75 patients (64%) with neoplasms and 43 patients (36%) with infectious or inflammatory lesions. Overall, 84% of the lesions in this series were benign. The ratio of neoplastic lesions to nonneoplastic swellings of the parotid gland of 1.74:1 in this pediatric population is noticeably different from that of most adult populations of 2.68:1.[15] Parotid swellings in children are therefore more likely to be infectious/inflammatory compared with parotid swellings in adults, which are more likely to be neoplastic.

Acute suppurative parotitis
Acute parotitis in children and infants (**Fig. 3**) is primarily caused by salivary stasis and the most common responsible organisms are *Staphylococcus aureus* and *Streptococcus viridans*. As with adults, treatment of acute parotitis in children is primarily medical and involves hydration, sialagogues, and gentle massaging of the gland. In severe cases, intravenous antibiotics are required and surgical drainage may be necessary.

Chronic recurrent parotitis
Chronic recurrent parotitis, also known as juvenile recurrent parotitis, is defined as recurrent parotid

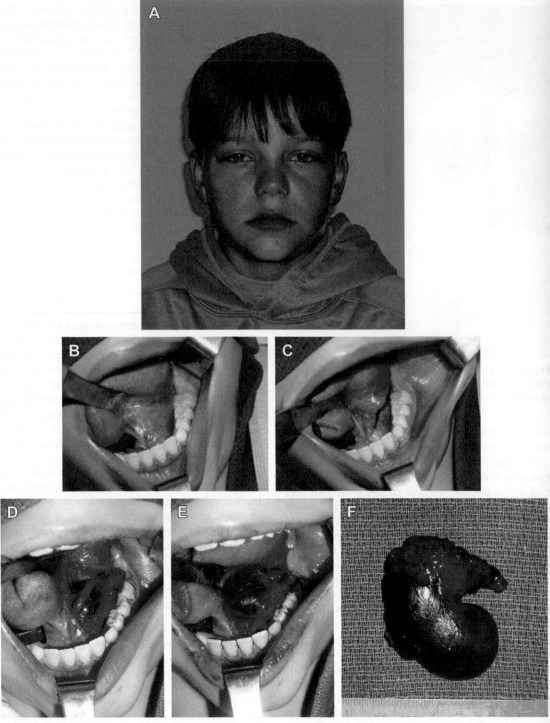

Fig. 2. A 10-year-old boy with a 2-week history of left neck swelling (*A*). Examination of the left floor of mouth identified a palpable lesion with a blue hue, suggestive of a ranula (*B*). Given the neck swelling, a clinical diagnosis of plunging ranula was made. The patient underwent surgical removal of the left sublingual gland and ranula. An incision was made in the left floor of mouth, lateral to the left Wharton duct opening (*C*). Dissection of the tissue bed resulted in the identification of the ranula deep to the Wharton duct (*D*). The ranula was carefully dissected free of the Wharton duct and lingual nerve (*E*) and the specimen was delivered (*F*). Final histopathology (*G*) confirmed the clinical diagnosis of ranula (H&E, original magnification × 20). The relationship of the lingual nerve and Wharton duct is noted superior to the mylohyoid muscle (*H*).

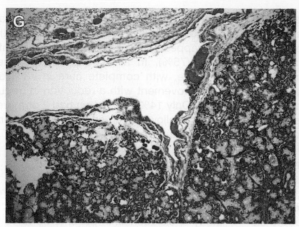

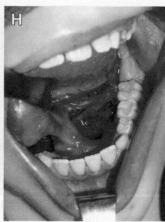

Fig. 2. (*continued*)

inflammation and is generally associated with non-obstructive sialectasia of the parotid gland.[16] Next to mumps, chronic recurrent parotitis is the most common inflammatory salivary gland disease in childhood and adolescence internationally.[17] The disease is more common in boys, characterized by recurring episodes of swelling and/or pain in the parotid gland, and is commonly accompanied by fever and malaise (**Fig. 4**). There is typically an absence of pus and the swelling lasts from several days to 2 weeks with spontaneous

resolution. The number of episodes varies, although the most common pattern is an attack every 3 to 4 months. The frequency rate peaks during the first year at school, and symptoms usually subside or completely disappear after puberty.[16] Clinical diagnosis can be confirmed by ultrasonography, which shows sialectasis or sialography showing sialectasis and ductal kinking.[18] Serum amylase can be a marker for the disease in the acute phase.[19]

Although the cause of chronic recurrent parotitis remains unclear, genetic, infectious (recurrent

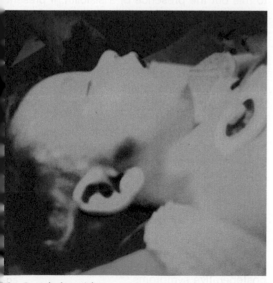

Fig. 3. A baby with an acute suppurative infection of the right parotid gland. It was thought that this infection represented hematogenous spread of a distant infection to an intraparotid lymph node. (*From* Carlson ER, Ord RA, editors. Salivary gland pathology – diagnosis and management. 2nd edition. Oxford (United Kingdom): Wiley; with permission.)

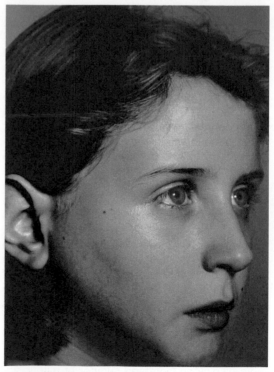

Fig. 4. A 6-year-old girl with recurrent right parotid swelling that indicates chronic recurrent parotitis.

viral), allergic, and immune-mediated causes are all possible. Maynard[20] proposed that a low salivary flow rate caused by dehydration results in a low-grade inflammation of the gland and duct epithelium. This inflammation in turn results in distortion and stricture of the distal ducts and metaplasia of the duct epithelium. Thereafter, the metaplasia results in excessive mucus secretion. These changes, along with a further reduction in salivary flow rate, then predispose the gland to recurrent inflammation. A reduced salivary flow rate may result from glandular damage caused by a primary infection in the gland. That notwithstanding, the reduced salivary flow rate may be the primary factor in the pathogenesis of the disease. Maynard[20] pointed out that the salivary flow rate was reduced in even the unaffected parotid gland in patients with unilateral disease.

Treatment of chronic recurrent parotitis is without universal acceptance in the international literature primarily because of the uncertainty regarding its cause as well as the rarity of the disease. As such, treatment of the acute episode has been centered on relief of pain and an attempt at preventing damage to the parenchyma of the gland. Antibiotics have been found to result in rapid decrease in swelling. Sialoendoscopy is also of benefit in the management of chronic recurrent parotitis in children. Hackett and colleagues[21] reported on 18 pediatric patients who underwent a total of 33 sialoendoscopic procedures on 27 glands. Chronic recurrent parotitis was the most frequent indication for surgery, with 12 children represented (67%) and 19 glands involved. Three patients had recurrent symptoms after the first sialoendoscopy. Eight patients required only 1 procedure to address their symptoms, 2 patients required 2 procedures, 1 patient required parotidectomy, and 1 patient was lost to follow-up. The investigators concluded that sialoendoscopy is both diagnostic and therapeutic for a clinical diagnosis of chronic recurrent parotitis. Shacham and colleagues[22] reported on 70 children with chronic recurrent parotitis and 5 adult patients who had chronic parotitis similar to the children. All patients underwent sialoendoscopy with lavage and dilatation and endoscopic injection of hydrocortisone into the gland. In 93% of patients a single endoscopic evaluation resulted in resolution of this disease and prevented its recurrence. In their comprehensive review of the literature on the use of sialoendoscopy in the management of juvenile recurrent parotitis, Canzi and colleagues[23] identified 10 research series that they included in their review with a total of 179 children, including 109 boys, and with an average age of 7.8 years. The most relevant diagnostic finding with sialoendoscopy was the white wall appearance of the duct with absent vascularity (75%). In all reports the treatment was effective, with complete cure in 78% of cases or improvement with a reduction in frequency of 22%. Only 14% of children had 2 or more procedures. Follow-up times for these reports were short, with a range of 4 to 36 months.

Acute submandibular sialadenitis and sialolithiasis

Acute submandibular sialadenitis is a rare condition in pediatric patients (**Fig. 5**). In their 30-year study of sialadenitis in patients up to 16 years of age, Kaban and colleagues[24] identified 49 patients requiring 67 hospitalizations. Four distinct types of sialadenitis were diagnosed, including 18 patients with acute suppurative parotitis, 14 patients with recurrent parotitis, 9 patients with chronic parotitis, and 8 patients with acute submandibular sialadenitis. Obstruction of the Wharton duct was the cause of all 8 cases of acute submandibular sialadenitis, 7 of which involved sialolithiasis, and 1 of which involved a congenital ductal stenosis. All patients with sialolithiasis underwent submandibular gland excision, and the 1 patient with congenital stenosis underwent a reconstructive duct procedure. As in adult patients, submandibular sialadenitis in pediatric patients should first be evaluated with radiographs to rule out the presence of a sialolith. If present, expedient removal should be undertaken (**Fig. 6**). Sialolithiasis in pediatric patients is very rare, accounting for only 3% of all sialolithiasis.[25] In adults, sialolithiasis occurs with an estimated prevalence of 12 per 1000 patients and a peak prevalence between 30 and 60 years of age. The youngest patient with sialolithiasis reported in the literature is a 2–year-old boy.[25,26] In a review of pediatric sialoliths versus adult sialoliths, Chung and colleagues[27] found that stones were more likely to be smaller and in the distal duct in children. They recommended careful bimanual palpation for diagnosis and intraoral stone removal in most children. Similar findings in radiological imaging of pediatric patients with salivary stones have been reported.[28] The long-term outcome for children who have intraoral stone removal is excellent, with 82.4% being without postoperative symptoms.[29]

An alternative to open retrieval of sialoliths is lithotripsy, which has been undertaken in children with sialolithiasis. In one series of 7 children, extracorporeal electromagnetic shock wave lithotripsy achieved complete stone disintegration in 5 cases, and in 2 cases a residual fragment less than 2 mm

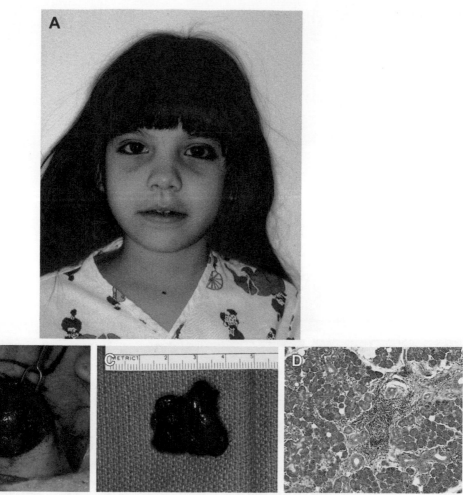

Fig. 5. A 7-year-old girl (*A*) with recurrent swellings of the left submandibular gland. Conservative measures were undertaken initially without success. She was therefore subjected to excision of the left submandibular gland (*B*, *C*). Histopathology identified mild sialadenitis of the submandibular gland (H&E, original magnification × 20) (*D*). (*From* Carlson ER, Ord RA, editors. Salivary gland pathology – diagnosis and management. 2nd edition. Oxford (United Kingdom): Wiley; with permission.)

was seen on ultrasonography imaging.[30] A mean of 5 sessions was required to achieve this result.[30] Sialoendoscopy has also been used both as a diagnostic and therapeutic procedure in children with salivary stones.[31]

If a sialolith is not identified, medical management should be performed, including proper hydration and empiric antibiotic therapy. Severe cases of sialadenitis (those cases in which questionable parental compliance exists) or immunocompromised patients require inpatient therapy involving intravenous antibiotics and fluids. Mild cases in otherwise healthy patients with effective parental support can be effectively managed on an outpatient basis. The development of chronic submandibular sialadenitis is not anticipated in pediatric patients as commonly occurs in adults.

NEOPLASTIC SALIVARY GLAND DISEASE

Salivary gland tumors are rare in children and include benign and malignant epithelial and mesenchymal neoplasms. A review of their incidence is noted in **Table 1**, which shows significant differences in the incidence and anatomic distribution of tumors in adult and pediatric populations. The 1991 AFIP data showed that children accounted for only 4.5% of all patients with salivary gland tumors. Mixed tumors, mucoepidermoid carcinomas, and acinic cell adenocarcinomas accounted for more than 92% of all epithelial tumors and about 77% of all tumors in this age group. In this series, and that of others,[1,6,32,33] mucoepidermoid carcinoma is the most common salivary gland malignancy in

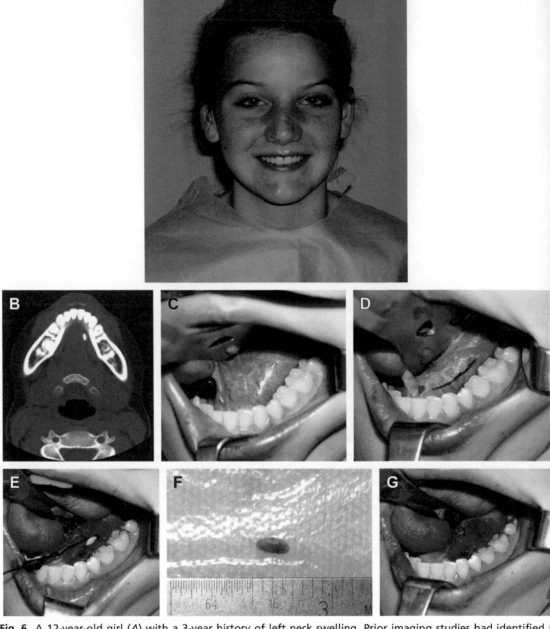

Fig. 6. A 12-year-old girl (*A*) with a 3-year history of left neck swelling. Prior imaging studies had identified a sialolith located in the left extraglandular Wharton duct (*B*). Another surgeon had unsuccessfully attempted a retrieval of the sialolith with a sialodochoplasty (*C*). The patient was prepared for sialolithotomy with transoral access (*D*). The Wharton duct was cannulated and the sialolith was able to be located (*E*) and removed (*F*). A sialodochoplasty was accomplished (*G*).

children. The mixed tumor is the most common benign salivary gland tumor in children in large series.[1,2] The benign and malignant epithelial salivary gland tumors together account for approximately 85% of all salivary gland tumors

reported in children.[2] The slight preponderance of benign tumors (55%) in pediatric patients is lower than the 63% incidence of benign salivary gland tumors in all patients in the AFIP data.[2] This observation that malignant tumors are more

Table 1
Comparison of the reported incidence of epithelial salivary gland neoplasms in pediatric and adult populations

Incidence	Pediatric Patients 3–4/Million/y	Adult Patients 80/Million/y
All salivary tumors (%)	5	90
Benign (%)	50	80
Malignant (%)	50	20
All salivary gland tumors occurring in the parotid gland (%)	85	82
Benign (%)	48	90
Malignant (%)	52	10
All salivary gland tumors occurring in the submandibular gland (%)	11	8
Benign (%)	33	67
Malignant (%)	67	33
All salivary gland tumors occurring in the sublingual gland (%)	3	1
Benign (%)	85	2
Malignant (%)	15	98
All salivary gland tumors occurring in the minor salivary glands (%)	1	8
Benign (%)	50	60
Malignant (%)	50	40

Adapted from Bradley PJ, Hartley B. Salivary gland neoplasms. In: Bradley PJ, Guntinas-Lichius O, editors. Salivary gland disorders and diseases: diagnosis and management. Stuttgart (Germany): Thieme; 2011. p. 94; with permission.

common than benign tumors in pediatric patients suggests that the pathogenesis of salivary gland tumors in pediatric patients might be different from that of adults. A genetic predisposition for cancer may be seen, because in one series 4 of 17 pediatric salivary cancers (23.5%) were second cancers occurring 6 to 9 years after the development and treatment of the first primary cancer.[34]

Epithelial Tumors

In the series of 494 total salivary gland tumors in children by Ellis and colleagues,[2] 422 (85%) were epithelial in nature and 72 (15%) were mesenchymal. This series included 271 benign tumors of which 210 (78%) were epithelial, and 223 malignant tumors of which 212 (95%) were epithelial. In these pediatric patients, pleomorphic adenoma was the most common tumor overall, accounting for 193 (39%) of the 494 pediatric tumors and 3.9% of all similar tumors occurring in all age groups owing to the greater frequency of the diagnosis of pleomorphic adenoma in adult patients. These 193 pleomorphic adenomas represented 92% of the 210 benign epithelial tumors and 71% of the total combined benign epithelial and benign mesenchymal tumors. Warthin tumor was the second most common benign epithelial tumor, accounting for only 5 cases (2.4% of benign epithelial tumors).

In their series of 80 salivary gland tumors in children, Lack and Upton[6] identified 25 epithelial tumors (31%), of which 10 were pleomorphic adenomas (40%), 6 were mucoepidermoid carcinomas (24%), and 5 were acinic cell carcinomas (20%). The pleomorphic adenomas were located in the parotid gland in 5 cases, in the submandibular gland in 4 cases, and in the soft palate in 1 case. In China, pleomorphic adenoma represented 91.45% of benign childhood tumors and mucoepidermoid carcinoma 47.1% of malignant tumors.[35]

Parotid tumors

In their review of the Salivary Gland Register from 1965 to 1984 at the University of Hamburg, Seifert and colleagues[36] reported on 9883 cases of salivary gland lesions, including 3326 neoplasms, 80 (2.4%) of which occurred in children. Fifty-seven (71%) of these tumors developed in the parotid gland. Pleomorphic adenoma accounted for virtually all of the benign pediatric neoplasms occurring in the parotid gland, with the Warthin tumor representing a minor contribution at this anatomic site. In 166 children with epithelial parotid tumors, 93 (55%) were benign and 73 (45%) were malignant.[37] In addition, these investigators pointed out that although the parotid gland is a less common site for salivary gland tumors in children compared with adults, there is a greater chance for malignancy in children in this site.

The work-up of a child with a parotid swelling does not differ significantly from that of an adult. Once inflammatory disease has been ruled out, a fine-needle aspiration biopsy of a discrete parotid mass in a child is useful to establish its cytologic character. Structural imaging is also valuable to establish the anatomic extent of the tumor. Superficial parotidectomy or partial superficial parotidectomy with facial nerve identification and preservation are the procedures of choice for pediatric parotid tumors (**Fig. 7**). Facial nerve sacrifice is only performed when preoperative palsy is noted to exist or when nerve invasion is appreciated intraoperatively. The facial nerve is more superficial in infants younger than 4 months of age compared with older children because of the lack of development of the mastoid process.[37] This anatomic difference in pediatric patients must be respected so as to maintain the integrity of the facial nerve during parotidectomy.

Submandibular gland tumors

As in adults, submandibular gland tumors are very uncommon in pediatric patients. Of 168 salivary gland tumors in the series of Krolls and colleagues,[1] submandibular gland tumors included 3 lymphomas, 4 mucoepidermoid carcinomas, and 10 benign tumors. Lack and Upton[6] identified 4 of 10 cases of pleomorphic adenoma occurring in the submandibular gland. In Castro and colleagues'[5] series of 38 major salivary gland tumors, 5 were noted to occur in the submandibular gland. These tumors included 4 cases of pleomorphic adenoma and 1 case of malignant mixed tumor. The treatment of benign submandibular gland tumors in children includes excision of the submandibular gland and tumor en bloc in an identical fashion to the management of these tumors in adult patients.

Minor salivary gland tumors

Minor salivary gland tumors in children are rare. Population studies have shown that only 5% of minor salivary gland tumors occur in children,

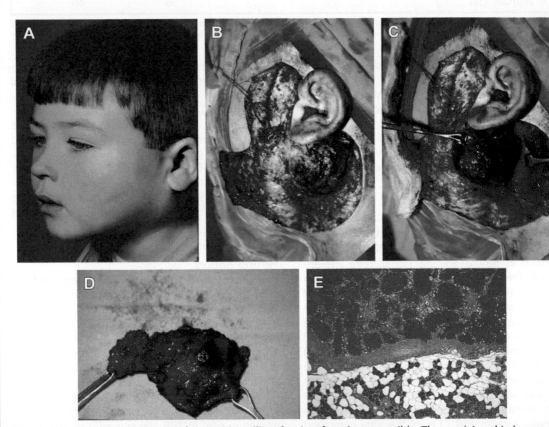

Fig. 7. A 3-year-old boy (*A*) with left parotid swelling that is soft and compressible. The overlying skin has a subtle blue hue that indicates a hemangioma. The angiogram supported this diagnosis. The patient underwent left superficial parotidectomy (*B, C*) and the specimen was delivered (*D*) Histopathology identified hemangioma (*E*). Hematoxylin and eosin, original magnification ×100. (*Courtesy of* [*E*] Dr Peter Sadow, Department of Pathology, Massachusetts General Hospital, Boston, MA; with permission.)

with a near equal distribution of benign and malignant tumors.[38] Preferred treatment of benign and malignant minor salivary gland tumors in children is identical to that in adults. The surgical management of benign palatal salivary gland tumors, like that of malignant salivary gland tumors, is identical to those surgeries performed in adult patients (**Fig. 8**). Specifically, the inclusion of the periosteum on the deep surface of the tumor provides effective cure of these benign tumors. The superiorly located maxillary bone need not be included with the tumor specimen. The exposed bone surface of the palate can be covered with local flaps or permitted to granulate and mucosalize in a tertiary fashion.

Mesenchymal Tumors

Mesenchymal salivary gland tumors are much more commonly noted in children than in adults. Ellis and colleagues[2] found 40 hemangiomas among 61 benign mesenchymal tumors (66%) and 72 benign and malignant mesenchymal tumors (56%). Lack and Upton[6] found 27 hemangiomas in their series of 80 pediatric salivary gland tumors (34%), which represented 49% of their 55 mesenchymal tumors.

Vascular tumors

Vascular salivary gland tumors in children typically occur in the parotid gland, are most commonly noted at or soon after birth, and are more frequent in girls.[6,37] In general, vascular tumors are classified as hemangioendotheliomas and hemangiomas. Hemangioendotheliomas occur in patients younger than 6 months of age, with rapid growth and aggressive behavior. Hemangiomas are slower growing processes that occur in older children. Krolls and colleagues[1] described hemangioendothelioma as an immature hemangioma. Such tumors are characterized by a unique tripartite growth cycle of proliferation, plateau, and involution. Although most involute without intervention, many require medical or surgical treatment. Krolls and colleagues[1] reported that the parotid gland was involved in 37 of their 39 vascular lesions. In Lack and Upton's[6] series of 27 cases of hemangioma, all of which occurred in the parotid gland, 19 occurred in female patients and 8 occurred in male patients.[6] A decided left-sided laterality was realized with a 5-times greater occurrence of the hemangioma of the left parotid gland compared with the right parotid gland. A median age of 4 months was noted in this series, with the oldest child being 16 months of age. Clinical findings typically include a soft, compressible mass with a bluish hue to the skin. Regression and involution of rapidly growing infantile

hemangioendotheliomas of the parotid gland have been reported,[39] although parotid lesions may be associated with slower involution or scarring.[40] Following involution, phleboliths may develop and can be seen radiographically in older children (**Fig. 9**).

Management of parotid hemangioendotheliomas has evolved as the natural history and behavior have become better understood. Radiation therapy was once used successfully for rapidly growing tumors in infants; however, the observation of late secondary malignancies in irradiated children has resulted in the abandonment of this modality of treatment. Surgical excision became the mainstay of treatment for many years and is occasionally still required. Excision of these lesions in infants and young children incurs a high risk for complications, including death, facial nerve palsy, and recurrence of the tumor. As such, most investigators now recommend nonoperative management for infants based on the anticipated spontaneous regression of these tumors.

In childhood hemangiomas the efficacy of systemic corticosteroid therapy is well documented[41,42] and interferon alfa-2a and alfa-2b have been used successfully.[43,44] However, a shift toward the use of β-blockers in infantile hemangiomas has occurred as a standard of care.[45] Propranolol is widely accepted to be a safer and better tolerated drug than oral corticosteroids. There is evidence that the use of propranolol is also distinguished from oral corticosteroids in its effectiveness in treating infants who are beyond the proliferative phase of growth. The proposed mechanism of action of propranolol includes rapid vasoconstriction of the lesion. Inhibition of angiogenesis by downregulation of proangiogenic growth factors, vascular endothelial growth factor, basic fibroblast growth factor, and matrix metalloproteinases 2 and 9 seems to correspond with growth arrest. In addition, the hastening of the induction of apoptosis of endothelial cells has been proposed to result in the stimulation of regression of infantile hemangiomas. Surgical resection is reserved for those tumors that do not respond to medical therapy.

Lymphatic malformations

Lack and Upton[6] reported 19 children with a diagnosis of lymphangioma involving salivary glands, which presented occasionally as a primary focus of involvement, but more commonly with more extensive involvement of juxtaglandular soft tissues and secondary encasement of the salivary gland (**Fig. 10**). These 19 lymphangiomas were the second most common mesenchymal tumor in their series, in which 27 cases of hemangioma

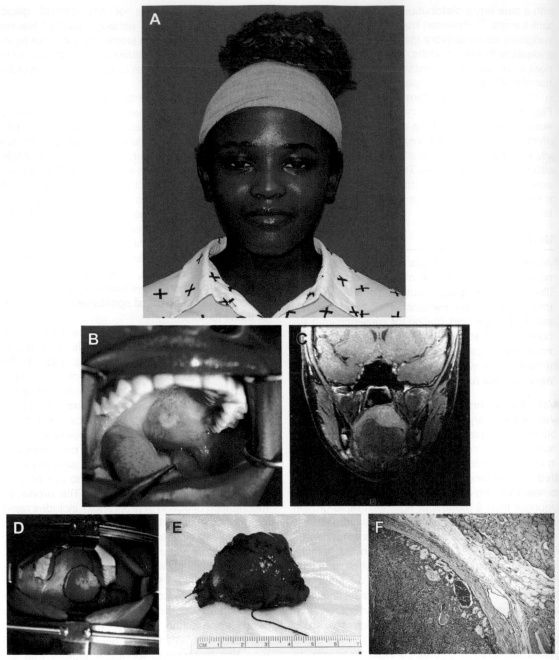

Fig. 8. A 12-year-old girl (*A*) with a long history of a slowly growing mass of the palate (*B*). Coronal T2-weighted MRI (*C*) identifies a hyperintense multilobulated mass consistent with a pleomorphic adenoma, which was confirmed by incisional biopsy. The patient underwent wide local excision of the mass (*D*) with sacrifice of the periosteum and a split-thickness dissection of the soft palate musculature as the deep anatomic barriers on the specimen (*E*). Final histopathology identified pleomorphic adenoma (H&E, original magnification × 10) (*F*). Coverage of the palatal defect (*G*) was accomplished with local flaps (*H*). (*Courtesy of* Dr John Caccamesse, Department of Oral and Maxillofacial Surgery, University of Maryland, Baltimore, Maryland; with permission.)

were most commonly noted. The lymphangiomas were 6 times more common in girls, with a median age of 6 years and equal distribution on each side of the neck. In their series of 494 pediatric salivary

gland tumors, Ellis and colleagues[2] identified only 5 cases of lymphangioma among 61 total benign mesenchymal tumors, which also included 40 cases of hemangioma.

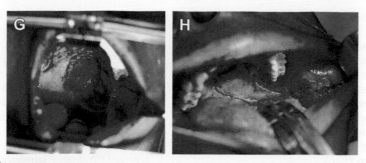

Fig. 8. (*continued*)

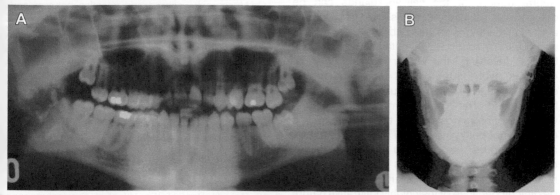

Fig. 9. An 18-year-old patient with calcifications superimposed over the right mandibular ramus on panoramic (*A*) and posterior-anterior (*B*) radiographs. The radiographs confirm the presence of phleboliths of the right parotid gland, which indicates a hemangioma of this gland.

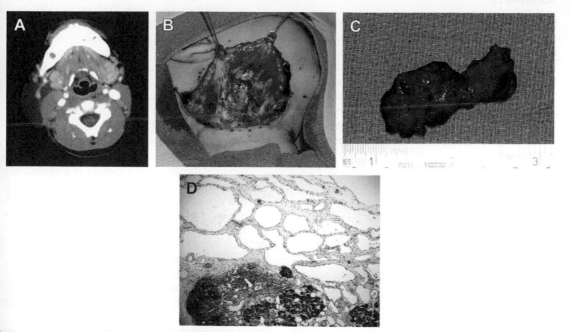

Fig. 10. CT scan (*A*) of an 11-month-old boy with a suspected lymphangioma of the right neck. The tumor is noted to be intimately involved with the right submandibular gland and parotid gland. Exploration of the neck (*B*) identified a large mass of these areas that was removed (*C*). Lymphangioma was confirmed by final histopathologic sections (*D*) (H&E, original magnification × 10).

Treatment recommendations of salivary lymphangioma have included observation, injection of sclerosing agents, and conservative surgery. Sclerosing agents are most successful in those lesions that have large cystic spaces. Surgical excision with preservation of the facial nerve in the case of a parotid lymphangioma is not likely to completely remove the abnormal lymphatic channels and microcysts. However, this debulking procedure proves to be clinically effective in controlling the disease.[37]

Neural tumors

Neural tumors of the salivary glands can be categorized as neurofibromas, neurilemmomas, and manifestations of neurofibromatosis.[37] Lack and Upton[6] reported 6 patients with neural tumors involving the major salivary glands, 4 tumors involving the parotid gland, and 1 case each involving the submandibular gland and sublingual gland. The most common clinical setting was neurofibromatosis, with the corresponding neural tumor being a plexiform neurofibroma. Ellis and colleagues[2] reported 10 neural tumors, 7 cases of neurofibroma, and 3 cases of schwannoma. Complete removal of neurofibromas can be difficult because of their highly infiltrative nature such that debulking with preservation of normal anatomy is preferred.

SUMMARY

Benign pediatric salivary gland lesions exist within a spectrum of nonneoplastic to neoplastic pathologic entities. However, their presence may negatively affect the young patient's appearance and function, necessitating expedient diagnosis and treatment with the realization of an acceptable result. Knowledge of this broad group of lesions as well as a scientifically valid approach to surgical or nonsurgical therapy represents an opportunity to this end.

REFERENCES

1. Krolls SO, Trodahl JN, Boyers RC. Salivary gland lesions in children. A survey of 430 cases. Cancer 1972;30:459–69.
2. Ellis GL, Auclair PL, Gnepp DR. Surgical pathology of the salivary glands. Chapter 9. Philadelphia: WB Saunders; 1991. p. 148–9.
3. Craver RD, Carr R. Paediatric salivary gland pathology. Diagn Histo 2012;18:373–80.
4. Ajike SO, Lakhoo K. Salivary gland diseases in children and adolescents. Available at: www.globalhelp.org/publicatons/books/help_pedsurgeryafrica39.pdf. Accessed April 2, 2015.
5. Castro EB, Huvos AG, Strong EW, et al. Tumors of the major salivary glands in children. Cancer 1972; 29:312–7.
6. Lack EE, Upton MP. Histopathologic review of salivary gland tumors in childhood. Arch Otolaryngol Head Neck Surg 1988;114:898–906.
7. Tasca RA, Clarke R. Inflammatory and infectious diseases of the salivary glands. Chapter 13. In: Bradley PJ, Guntinas-Lichius O, editors. Salivary gland disorders and diseases: diagnosis and management. Stuttgart (Germany): Georg Thieme Verlag; 2011. p. 110–20.
8. Hayashida AM, Zerbinatti DCZ, Balducci I, et al. Mucus extravasation and retention phenomena: a 24-year study. BMC Oral Health 2010;10:1–4.
9. Bhargava N, Agarwal P, Sharma N, et al. An unusual presentation of oral mucocele in infant and its review. Case Rep Dentistry 2014;2014: 723130.
10. Syebele K, Butow KW. Oral mucoceles and ranulas may be part of initial manifestations of HIV infection. Aids Res Hum Retroviruses 2010;26:1075–8.
11. Pandit RT, Park AH. Management of pediatric ranula. Otolaryngol Head Neck Surg 2002;127:115–8.
12. Zhi K, Wen Y, Ren W, et al. Management of infant ranula. Int J Pediatr Otorhinolaryngol 2008;72:823–6.
13. Seo JH, Park JJ, Kim HY, et al. Surgical management of intraoral ranulas in children: an analysis of 17 pediatric cases. Int J Pediatr Otorhinolaryngol 2010;74:202–5.
14. Orvidas LJ, Kasperbauer JL, Lewis JE, et al. Pediatric parotid masses. Arch Otolaryngol Head Neck Surg 2000;126:177–84.
15. Gallia LJ, Johnson JT. The incidence of neoplastic versus inflammatory disease in major salivary gland masses diagnosed by surgery. Laryngoscope 1981; 91:512–6.
16. Chitre VV, Premchandra DJ. Recurrent parotitis. Arch Dis Child 1997;77:359–63.
17. Ellies M, Laskawi R. Diseases of the salivary glands in infants and adolescents. Head Face Med 2010;6:1–7.
18. Nahlieli O, Shacham R, Shlesinger M, et al. Juvenile recurrent parotitis: a new method of diagnosis and treatment. Pediatrics 2004;114:9–12.
19. Saarinen R, Kolho KL, Davidkin I, et al. The clinical picture of juvenile parotitis in a prospective setup. Acta Paediatr 2013;102:177–81.
20. Maynard JD. Recurrent parotid enlargement. Br J Surg 1965;52:784–9.
21. Hackett AM, Baranano CF, Reed M, et al. Sialoendoscopy for the treatment of pediatric salivary gland disorders. Arch Otolaryngol Head Neck Surg 2012; 138:912–5.
22. Shacham R, Droma EB, London D, et al. Long-term experience with endoscopic diagnosis and treatment of juvenile recurrent parotitis. J Oral Maxillofac Surg 2009;67:162–7.

23. Canzi P, Occhini A, Pagella F, et al. Sialendoscopy in juvenile recurrent parotitis; a review of the literature. Acta Otorhinolaryngol Ital 2013;33:367–73.

24. Kaban LB, Mulliken JB, Murray JE. Sialadenitis in childhood. Am J Surg 1978;135:570–6.

25. Kim DH, Song WS, Kim YJ, et al. Parotid sialolithiasis in a two-year old boy. Korean J Pediatr 2013;56:451–5.

26. Liu NM, Rawal J. Submandibular sialolithiasis in a child. Arch Dis Child 2013;98:407.

27. Chung MK, Jeong HS, Ko MH, et al. Pediatric sialolithiasis: what is different from adult sialolithiasis? Int J Pediatr Otorhinolaryngol 2007;71:787–91.

28. Salerno S, Giordano J, La Tona G, et al. Pediatric sialolithiasis distinctive characteristics in radiological imaging. Minerva Stomatol 2011;60:435–41.

29. Woo SH, Jang JY, Park GY, et al. Long-term outcome of intraoral submandibular stone removal in children as compared to adults. Laryngoscope 2009;119:116–20.

30. Ottaviani F, Marchisio P, Arisi E, et al. Extra corporeal shockwave lithotripsy for salivary calculi in pediatric patients. Acta Otolaryngol 2001;121:873–6.

31. Nahieli O, Ekiav E, Hasson O, et al. Pediatric sialolithiasis. Oral Surg Oral Med Oral Pathol Oral Radiol Endod 2000;90:709–12.

32. Laikui L, Hongwei L, Hongbing J, et al. Epithelial salivary gland tumors of children and adolescents in west China population: a clinicopathologic study of 79 cases. J Oral Pathol Med 2008;37:201–5.

33. Yoshida EJ, Garcia J, Eisele DW, et al. Salivary gland malignancies in children. Int J Ped Otorhinolaryngol 2014;78:174–8.

34. Chiaravali S, Guzzo M, Bisogno G, et al. Salivary gland carcinomas in children and adolescents: The Italian TREP project experience. Pediatr Blood Cancer 2014;61:1961–8.

35. Fang OG, Shi S, Li ZN, et al. Epithelial salivary gland tumors in children; a twenty five year experience of 122 patients. Int J Pediatr Otorhinolaryngol 2013;77:1252–4.

36. Seifert G, Okabe H, Caselitz J. Epithelial salivary gland tumors in children and adolescents. Analysis of 80 cases (Salivary Gland Register 1965-1984). ORL J Otorhinolaryngol Relat Spec 1986;48:137–49.

37. Ord RA. Salivary gland tumors in children. In: Kaban LB, Troulis MJ, editors. Pediatric oral and maxillofacial surgery. Philadelphia: Saunders; 2004. p. 202–11.

38. Galer C, Santillan AA, Chelius D, et al. Minor salivary gland malignancies in the pediatric population. Head Neck 2012;34:1648–51.

39. Scarcella JV, Dykes ER, Anderson R. Hemangiomas of the parotid gland. Plast Reconstr Surg 1965;36:38–47.

40. Drolet BA, Esterly NB, Frieden IJ. Hemangiomas in children. N Engl J Med 1999;341:173–81.

41. Gangopadhyay AN, Sinha CK, Gopal SC, et al. Role of steroids in childhood haemangioma: a 10-years review. Int Surg 1997;82:49–51.

42. Enjolras O, Rich MC, Merland JJ, et al. Management of alarming hemangiomas in infants: a review of 25 cases. Pediatrics 1990;25:491–8.

43. Ezekowitz RAB, Mulliken JB, Folkman J. Interferon alfa-2a therapy for life-threatening hemangiomas of infancy. N Engl J Med 1992;326:1456–63.

44. Soumekh B, Adams GL, Shapiro RS. Treatment of head and neck hemangiomas with recombinant interferon alpha-2b. Ann Otol Rhinol Laryngol 1996;105:201–6.

45. Puttgen KB. Diagnosis and management of infantile hemangiomas. Pediatr Clin North Am 2014;61:383–402.

Pediatric Salivary Gland Malignancies

Robert A. Ord, DDS, MD, FRCS, MS, MBA[a],*, Eric R. Carlson, DMD, MD[b]

KEYWORDS

- Pediatric malignant salivary gland tumors • Mucoepidermoid carcinoma • Parotid gland tumors

KEY POINTS

- Salivary gland neoplasms are rare in children, representing less than 5% of salivary malignancies.
- Malignant tumors are more frequent in children than adults, representing 40% to 60% of pediatric salivary neoplasms.
- Most pediatric salivary malignancies are epithelial tumors.
- Malignant salivary gland tumors are extremely rare in patients younger than 10 years of age.
- The parotid gland is the most common site, and the mucoepidermoid carcinoma is the most common histopathologic type.
- Survival and outcomes are better in children than adults.
- Surgery is the foundation of management. Radiation and chemotherapy have to be used in selected cases with care because of the occurrence of secondary malignant salivary neoplasms induced by these therapies.

INTRODUCTION

It is difficult to make definitive statements regarding salivary gland malignancies in children, as these are rare tumors. Head and neck cancers comprise approximately 3% of all malignancies, and salivary cancers comprise 3% of head neck cancers. Literature reviews conclude that pediatric cases of salivary cancer represent only 5% of all salivary cancers.[1] Because of their rarity and their heterogeneity, there are few large published series to review. In addition, when seeking to document the incidence of these tumors, many older series include nonneoplastic disease of the salivary glands as well as tumors. Finally, there is little agreement between authors as to what constitutes a pediatric patient, with younger than 14 years and up to younger than 20 years all being defined as pediatric.

Another conflicting variable is the fact that histologic classification of salivary glands has changed significantly in the last 50 years with the inclusion of newly recognized entities such as polymorphous low-grade adenocarcinoma and epimyoepithelial carcinoma. This makes interpretation of older studies difficult regarding the incidence of the different tumor types.

In order to try and keep the data as coherent as possible, the authors have therefore primarily used papers published since 2000 for this article, although older classic papers with large numbers have been cited as baseline references and to illustrate some specific points.

DEMOGRAPHICS

Although the Armed Forces Institute of Pathology (AFIP) published a large series of pediatric salivary

a Department of Oral and Maxillofacial Surgery, Baltimore College of Dental Surgery, University of Maryland and the Greenbaum Cancer Institute, Suite 1402, 650, West Baltimore Street, Baltimore, MD 21201, USA;
b Department of Oral and Maxillofacial Surgery, University of Tennessee Medical Center, 1930 Alcoa Highway, Suite 335, Knoxville, Tennessee 37920, USA
* Corresponding author.
E-mail address: rord@umm.edu

Oral Maxillofacial Surg Clin N Am 28 (2016) 83–89
http://dx.doi.org/10.1016/j.coms.2015.07.007
1042-3699/16/$ – see front matter © 2016 Elsevier Inc. All rights reserved

cases (430) in 1972,[2] this is a flawed study for determining incidence of pediatric neoplasms, as despite the large total number of 9993 lesions, the paper does not define how many were truly neoplastic. The study identified 430 salivary gland lesions in children younger than the age of 15 years, but only 168 lesions represented salivary gland tumors. Fifty-four of these were malignant (47% of pediatric salivary tumors), 35 of which were epithelial tumors; 6 tumors were mesenchymal. Six tumors were reticuloepithelial; 5 undifferentiated, and 2 tumors were metastatic. The most common malignancy was mucoepidermoid carcinoma (MECA) (20 cases), accounting for 5% of all MECAs accessioned by the AFIP. The most common site was parotid (14 cases), followed by submandibular and minor glands. There was an equal sex ratio, and the peak age was 10 years (although this study defined pediatric as under 15 years of age), the youngest being 1 year. The second most common tumor was acinic cell carcinoma (12 cases). Although this is an old study, it does show that pediatric salivary tumors are rare; there is a high percentage of malignant salivary neoplasms in children (almost 50%), and most are epithelial neoplasms. The parotid is the most common site; MECA is the most common malignant salivary tumor seen in children, and lesions are less frequent under the age of 10 years. These conclusions are largely supported by later studies with only minor differences in results from subsequent publications.

One other older paper by Ellis in 1991[3] reviewed 494 pediatric salivary tumors in patients younger than 17 years. Two hundred twenty-three tumors were malignant (45%), with 212 tumors (95%) being malignant epithelial tumors; the rest were malignant mesenchymal tumors, with MECA being the most common (123 cases, 55% of all malignant tumors). More recent studies do not have such long series of patients but do have more up-to-date histopathologic classifications.

Ribeiro Kde and colleagues[4] in a study from Brazil reported 38 cases of epithelial neoplasms of salivary glands under the age of 19 years with a mean age of 11.8 years and a female preponderance of 1.9:1. Twenty-seven of their patients had malignant tumors (71%); 65.8% of cases were located in the parotid, and 17 cases (63% of all malignancies) were MECA.

Sultan and colleagues[5] reviewed only malignant tumors in children from US SEER (Surveillance, Epidemiology and End Results) data. They reported 263 children under the age of 19 years, who comprised 2% of all salivary gland malignancies. This represents an annual incidence of 0.8 cases per million in children/adolescents.

Fifty-eight percent of their series were female; the parotid gland was the most common site, and 84% of the malignancies were MECAs or acinic cell carcinomas.

In 2006, Guzzo and colleagues[6] from Italy reviewed 52 cases of salivary epithelial neoplasms in children ages 4 to 18 years. Only 29% of cases were malignant; major glands were most affected, 79% in the parotid, and 80% of malignant tumors were MECAs.

A German paper (Muenscher and colleagues 2009[7]) reviewed children 14 years and younger and reported 211 neoplasms, of which 159 were malignant (75.3%). Of these tumors, 80.5% were epithelial, with the parotid and submandibular gland being the most common sites. Surprisingly, in this series epithelial–myoepithelial carcinomas (28%), carcinomas of the salivary duct (23%) were the most common, with MECA only found in 14%.

In contrast, there have been 3 studies from China in the last 6 years, and although they again have found the parotid as the most common site with MECA as the most common malignancy, there has been a much higher percentage of benign tumors in these pediatric cases. In 2008 Laikui and colleagues[8] reported 79 salivary tumors in children younger than 18 years old, with 24.1% of tumors being malignant, while in 2013, Deng and colleagues[9] reported 119 pediatric patients younger than 19 years with salivary neoplasms with 26.9% of tumors malignant; also in 2013 Fang and colleagues[10] reported 122 patients younger than 19 years with 13.9% of tumors being malignant.

It can be concluded that pediatric salivary cancers are rare, less than 5% of all salivary cancers with the overwhelming majority representing as epithelial neoplasms. There are a small minority of mesenchymal tumors that will be mentioned in this article. The percentage of malignant salivary gland tumors compared with benign is about 40% to 60% in children, which is much more frequent than in adults. Most tumors occur above the age of 10 years, and there is a slight propensity for females. The parotid is the most common site, and MECA is the most common tumor. In the Chinese population, malignant salivary tumors are seen less frequently in children, and their distribution is similar to that seen in adults.

ETIOLOGY

As is the case for adult salivary gland neoplasms, the etiology for the vast majority of salivary gland neoplasms in children is unknown. The Epstein Barr virus (EBV) has been reported as an mplication in the etiology of undifferentiated carcinomas, with high incidence in Inuit populations and lymphoepithelial salivary carcinomas. This association has been reported in pediatric salivary carcinomas.[11] In a paper from St. Jude Children's Research Hospital with 13 cases of salivary cancer 7 MECA), latent EBV infection was identified using n situ hybridization (ISH) technique.

Another etiologic factor in children is exposure o radiation or chemotherapy for other childhood cancers giving rise to later secondary induced salivary neoplasms. Initially this was felt to be a problem with radiation therapy only, particularly in the reatment of leukemia/lymphoma in children and giving rise to secondary mucoepidermoid carcinomas. In 2006, Védrine and colleagues[12] reported 18 MECAs in children younger than 20 years old in a multi-institutional French study. Eleven of these patients had been treated with radiation and/or chemotherapy, 4 for lymphoid leukemia, 3 for lymphoma, 2 for brain tumors, 1 sarcoma, and 1 retinoblastoma. In 2007, Miyatima and colleagues[13] reviewed the literature on MECA of the parotid gland following treatment for ymphoblastic leukemia and found 14 cases. Although 11 cases had radiation, there were three patients who had received chemotherapy without radiation. In the last 7 years, cases of childhood sarcoma[14] and neuroblastoma[15] treated with only chemotherapy have also been reported to develop MECA of the parotid.

In a systematic review of the literature in 2011,[16] 23 articles were entered into the study documenting 58 patients who developed MECA following previous chemotherapy and/or radiotherapy. Fourteen patients were treated only with radiation therapy, 14 with chemotherapy alone, and 30 patients with a combination of chemotherapy and radiation. The most common initial diagnosis was lymphoblastic leukemia (18 cases), followed by acne (9 cases), and Hodgkin lymphoma (6 cases). The latent time for developing MECA was 7.9 years for patients treated with radiation plus or minus chemotherapy but 27.2 years for radiation therapy alone. Obviously children who are treated at a very young age with chemotherapy plus or minus radiation and have a short latent time will develop their MECA when still in the pediatric age cohort. However, secondary MECA with a longer latent time will present in adulthood.

MANAGEMENT AND OUTCOME

The management of salivary gland cancer in children is based on surgical resection the same as for adults. Although salivary cancer is comparatively more common in children than in adults, it does appear to have a better overall prognosis in children. In a study from 2011 using SEER data,[17] 763 patients were identified younger than 30 years old. Survival was 100% for patients younger than 1 year, but this represented only 1 case. Relative 5-year survival was 50% in patients 1 to 4 years old, 87.2% among 5- to 9-year-olds, 97% in 10- to 14-year-olds and 95% in patients between the ages of 15 and 19 years.

In examining MECAs in children younger than 18 years old, 49 patients were documented, 49% of tumors in the parotid and 35% of tumors in minor salivary glands of the oral cavity.[18] Regional disease was found in 24% of cases. In this series, 100% of patients underwent surgery, and 22% had radiation therapy. Overall survival at 5 years was 98%, and at 10 years it was 94%. Ten percent of the cases developed recurrence. The authors concluded that MECA in children carried a favorable prognosis and can be treated with surgery alone in most cases. The following section will discuss the management of major salivary gland cancer and minor salivary gland cancer separately.

Management and Outcomes for Major Salivary Gland Cancers

In Sultan and colleagues[5] database review of SEER for major salivary gland malignancies in children, 88% of children/adolescents had oncologic surgery for their parotid gland malignancies. In 128 pediatric parotid tumors, 17 (13%) had excisional biopsy, 53 (41%) subtotal parotidectomy, and 51 (40%) total or radical parotidectomy. Of 74 patients, 21 had no neck dissection; 19 patients had 1 to 3 nodes removed, and 27 patients had removal of at least 4 nodes (36.5%). Only 27% of the pediatric cohort received adjuvant radiation, whereas 51% of adults were given radiation, which was highly significant ($p < .001$). Five-year overall survival was 95% plus or minus 1.5% for children/adolescents and 59% for adults, which was highly significant ($p < .001$). When the authors analyzed the factors that contributed to this survival advantage in children, they identified a number of significant differences between the cohorts. The pediatric tumors were more localized with less local extension or regional metastases (76% vs 50%, $p < .001$). In addition, pediatric tumors were much more likely to be well or moderately differentiated (88% vs 49% $p < .001$). Also, although the most common tumor for both cohorts was MECA, the percentage of other histologies was different, with MECA and acinic cell carcinoma comprising 83.6% of tumors in children and 35.4% in adults. The reduced number of high-grade, advanced stage tumors in children, as well as the effects of radiation on facial growth and inducing second cancers is probably the reason for radiation being used significantly less often in the pediatric cohort.

In a single-institution series from the MD Anderson Center of Pediatric Cancer in major salivary glands, 61 patients were studied.[19] Eighty-three percent of tumors arose in the parotid gland, with almost half (46%) representing MECA. Lymphatic metastasis was diagnosed in 37%, and 65% of the cohort had already been treated at another institution; however, more than 75% underwent surgical resection at MD Anderson. A total of 45% of patients received radiation therapy. Overall 5-year survival was 93%, and 26% of patients were diagnosed with a recurrence. Risk factors predicting adverse outcome were tumor grade, margin status, and neural involvement. The authors felt that radiation therapy was beneficial for locoregional control of disease.

Chiaravalli and colleagues 2014[20] described 17 pediatric patients with salivary cancer, 14 cases occurring in the parotid. Most were low grade, with favorable presentation and low stage as documented in other studies. All patients had primary surgery, although only 9 of 17 had negative margins. Adjuvant radiation therapy was given to 6 patients (35%). Only 1 patient died in this series.

Interestingly, those children who presented with secondary MECA induced by radiation plus or minus chemotherapy also had good outcomes. Surgery was the most common treatment followed by surgery with postoperative radiation therapy, and 2- and 5-year overall survival rates were 98% and 93.4%, respectively. The 2- and 5-year locoregional control rates were 97.7% and 92.5%, respectively.[16]

The submandibular gland as a subsite is not clearly defined in most studies, and the paucity of cases and lack of data do not allow any definitive statements to be made regarding management. **Fig. 1** illustrates a complex and possibly unique case of submandibular gland malignancy in a child (see **Fig. 1**).

Management and Outcomes for IntraOral Minor Salivary Gland Cancers

Minor salivary gland tumors are uncommon but comprise the second most common site in children after parotid tumors.[1] In a series of 426 intraoral benign and malignant minor salivary gland tumors, only 16 tumors (3.8%) occurred in patients under the age of 19 years.[21] In this series, there were 181 malignant tumors, and of these 3 tumors (1.7%) occurred in patients younger than 19 years. In a study of 311 intraoral benign and malignant salivary gland tumors from Thailand 18 (5.9%) cases were younger than 19 years old. Malignant tumors were found in 164 patients, and 9 (5.5%) patients were younger than 19 years.[22]

Because of the rarity of these cases, there are very few treatment/outcome analyses for minor salivary gland tumors in pediatric patients. There is a single-institution report on minor salivary gland tumors in patients younger than 18 years from MD Anderson with 35 cases, 20 of which were in the oral cavity (57.1%).[23] The authors recommend surgical resection with negative margins giving excellent results with low- to intermediate-grade tumors and early stage cancers. Despite

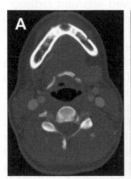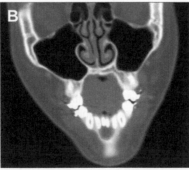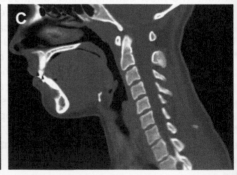

Fig. 1. (*A–C*) The patient is a 15-year-old girl who had removal of a submandibular gland tumor at age 11 years, which showed a benign pleomorphic adenoma. Three years later, a radiolucency was noted on a panoramic film. The figure shows the axial (*A*), coronal (*B*), and sagittal cuts (*C*) of a subsequent computed tomography (CT) scan, which confirms a benign-appearing radiolucency (differential diagnosis a cyst or giant cell lesion) in the midline of the mandible below the apices of the incisors. The lesion was enucleated, and the histology was consistent with benign pleomorphic adenoma. Final diagnosis in this case was a malignant pleomorphic adenoma, histopathologically benign metastasizing pleomorphic adenoma.

multimodal therapy, high-grade cancers did poorly. Five-year overall survival and disease-specific survival were 89.35% and 88.4%, respectively. There were 4 patients who recurred, and this was significantly associated with positive margins, advanced stage and high grade. Children in this series had 88.6% low-grade tumors, 75.6% early stage disease, and 62.9% of tumors were MECA.

In an unpublished series from the University of Maryland, 279 minor salivary gland tumors of the oral cavity were seen from 1989 to 2014; 12 (4.3%) tumors were in children younger than 19 years of age. Ten of 209 of these tumors were malignant (4.8%, **Table 1**). The palate was the most common site for malignant tumors (70%), and low- to intermediate-grade tumors comprised 90% of tumors, while stage 1 and 2 disease also represented 90% of tumors (**Fig. 2**).

There has been controversy regarding the management of low- to intermediate-grade MECA of the palate and whether bone resection of the palate or maxilla is required if there is no clinical or radiologic evidence of bone invasion. In 1972, Eversole and colleagues[24] showed a 0% recurrence rate with wide local resection and only resecting bone if it was involved. Despite these results, in 1981, Olson and colleagues[25] advocated palatal bone resection for all MECAs. In 1985, Conley and colleagues[26] reported 4 pediatric cases treated by composite resection with no recurrence. These patients had previously been treated with wide local excision, and no tumor was found in the reresection specimens. In 2002, a similar series of 4 pediatric patients with low-grade MECA of the palate treated by wide local

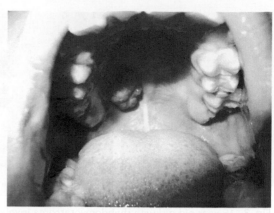

Fig. 2. Intraoral photograph shows a T1N0M0 stage 1 low grade MECA of the palate in an 11-year-old Hispanic girl. Managed by wide local excision with conservation of the palatal bone. Patient has no recurrence 4 years and 7 months postoperatively.

excision and no bone resection was reported by one of the authors.[27] Zero recurrence was seen with no morbidity. A larger series of 18 adult cases also from the University of Maryland confirmed these findings.[28]

CONCLUSION FOR OUTCOMES

Salivary cancers in children have better survival than adults. This is related to the fact that low and intermediate tumors are more common in children; the tumors present at an early stage and are more localized and less likely to have regional disease. Surgery is the primary treatment, and multimodality therapy is used only for patients with high

Table 1
Pediatric minor salivary gland tumors at the University of Maryland 1989 – 2014

Patient #	Gender	Age	Race	Site	Histologic Type	Stage
1	F	13	W	Palate	Low grade MECA	T1N0M0
2	F	16	W	Soft Palate	Int grade MECA	T2N0M0
3	M	16	B	Palate	Low grade MECA	T1N0M0
4	M	11	W	Palate	Low grade MECA	T1N0M0
5	F	13	W	Buccal	PLGA	T1N0M0
6	F	16	H	Max Alveolus	ACC	T4N0M0
7	F	17	W	Palate	Pleomorphic adenoma	—
8	F	9	W	Buccal	Low-grade mucous-producing adeno CA	T1N0M0
9	F	16	W	Palate	Low-grade MECA	T2N0M0
10	M	11	W	Palate	Low-grade MECA	T2N0M0
11	F	13	H	Palate	Low-grade MECA	T1N0M0
12	M	19	B	Palate	Pleomorphic adenoma	—

Abbreviations: ACC, adenoid cystic carcinoma; Adeno CA, adenocarcinoma; MECA, mucoepidermoid carcinoma; PLGA, polymorphous low grade adenocarcinoma.

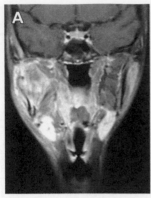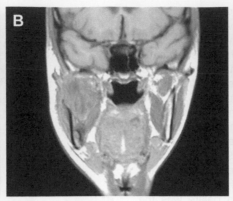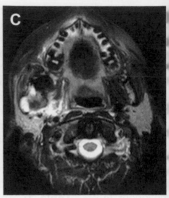

Fig. 3. 15-year-old girl with rhabdomyosarcoma involving mandible, masticator space and deep lobe of parotid. Mother refused primary surgery and patient failed protocol chemotherapy plus radiation. Magnetic resonance (MR) shows: (*A*) MR coronal view rhabdomyosarcoma of masticator space involving mandible, medial pterygoid and deep lobe of parotid. (*B*) MR coronal view shows extension to skull base (parameningeal type). (*C*) MR axial view shows involvement of pterygoid plates and deep lobe of the parotid. She underwent vertical compartment resection with fibular reconstruction. She recurred 1 year after salvage surgery, and failed further chemotherapy and died of local disease.

risk due to large, advanced-stage tumors, positive margins after surgery, or high histologic grade. Secondary MECA tumors seem to do as well as tumors with no obvious etiology. There is much less evidence for the treatment of minor salivary tumors compared with parotid malignancies in children.

Patients younger than 10 years seem to have a worse survival (relative 5-year survival 50% in patients 1–4 years old[17]), and this may be related to higher-grade malignancies under the age of 10 years.[29] Grade is the strongest indicator for survival for children with MECA, with 100% overall survival at 5 years for low to intermediate tumors compared with 50% for high-grade tumors.[23] This correlates with Hicks' and Flaitz's basic research work on proliferation markers in MECA in children.[30]

NONEPITHELIAL SALIVARY TUMORS IN CHILDREN

Although lymphomas and secondary metastatic tumors do occur in the salivary glands in children, most of these entities are reported as single cases or very small series. It is really only mesenchymal tumors and in particular rhabdomyosarcomas that have enough reported cases to draw any conclusions as to management. In Sultan's SEER analysis,[5] 263 children with epithelial neoplasms of the salivary glands were identified, and 17 additional cases of mesenchymal cancers (16 parotid) were also found. Fourteen of the seventeen cases were diagnosed as rhabdomyosarcoma. In 2001 the Intergroup Rhabdomyosarcoma Study Group reported on parotid rhabdomyosarcoma in

children.[31] They identified 62 patients with rhabdomyosarcoma in the parotid region, 30 of whom had invasion of a parameningeal site. Half of the nonparameningeal cohort had group 1 or 2 tumors, none in the parameningeal group, and group 3 tumors were the most common in both cohorts. One hundred percent of patients received radiation therapy and patients in the parameningeal cohort received intensified radiation and chemotherapy. The 5-year failure-free survival rate was 81%, and the 5-year survival rate was 84%. There was zero mortality in group 1 and 2 tumors and no difference between the 2 cohorts in survival. The authors concluded that the IRS (Intergroup Rhabdomyosarcoma Study Group) protocols were highly effective for treatment of rhabdomyosarcomas in the parotid region, even for parameningeal cases with intensified therapy. **Fig. 3** illustrates a pediatric rhabdomyosarcoma in the parotid region that failed chemotherapy and radiation.

REFERENCES

1. Yoshida EJ, García J, Eisle DW, et al. Salivary gland malignancies in children. Int J Pediatr Otorhinolaryngol 2014;78:174–8.
2. Krolls SO, Trodahl JN, Boyers RC. Salivary gland lesions in children. A survey of 430 cases. Cancer 1972;30:459–69.
3. Ellis GL, Auclair PL, Gnepp DR. Surgical pathology of the salivary glands. Philadelphia: WB Saunders Co; 1991. p. 148–9. Chapter 9.
4. Ribeiro Kde C, Kowalski LP, Saba LM, et al. Epithelial salivary gland neoplasms in children and

adolescents: a forty-four –year experience. Med Pediatr Oncol 2002;39:594–600.

5. Sultan I, Rodriguez-galindo C, Al-Sharabati S, et al. Salivary gland carcinomas in children and adolescents: a population based study with comparison to adult cases. Head Neck 2011;33(10):1476–81.

6. Guzzo M, Ferrari A, Mrcon I, et al. Salivary gland neoplasms in children: the experience of the Istituto Nazionale Tumori of Milan. Pediatr Blood Cancer 2006;46(6):806–10.

7. Meunscher A, Diegel T, Jaehne M, et al. Benign and malignant salivary gland diseases in children. A retrospective study of 549 cases from the salivary gland registry, Hamburg. Auris Nasus Larynx 2009; 36:326–31.

8. Laikui L, Hongwei W, Hongbing J, et al. Epithelial salivary gland tumors and adolescents in west China population: a clinicopathologic study of 79 cases. J Oral Pathol Med 2008;37:201–5.

9. Deng R, Huang X, Hao J, et al. Salivary gland neoplasms in children. J Craniofac Surg 2013;24(2): 511–3.

10. Fang QG, Shi S, Li ZN, et al. Epithelial salivary gland tumors in children: a twenty-five year experience of 122 patients. Int J Pediatr Otorhinolaryngol 2013; 77(8):1252–4.

11. Venkateswaran L, Gan YJ, Sixbey JW, et al. Epstein-Barr virus infection in salivary gland tumors in children and young adults. Cancer 2000;89(2):463–6.

12. Védrine PO, Coffinet L, Teman S, et al. Mucoepidermoid carcinoma of salivary glands in the pediatric age group: 18 clinical cases, including 11 second malignant neoplasms. Head Neck 2006; 28(9):827–33.

13. Miyatima Y, Ogawa A, Kuno K, et al. Mucoepidermoid carcinoma of the parotid gland as a secondary malignancy developed ten years after chemotherapy for childhood acute lymphoblastic leukemia. Rinsho Ketsueki 2007;48(6):491–4.

14. Rutigliano DN, Meyers P, Ghossein RA, et al. Mucoepidermoid carcinoma as a second malignancy in pediatric sarcoma. J Pediatr Surg 2007;42(7):E9–12.

15. Blatt J, Zdanski C, Scanga L, et al. Mucoepidermoid carcinoma of the parotid as a second malignancy after chemotherapy in a child with neuroblastoma. J Pediatr Hematol Oncol 2013;35(5):399–401.

16. Verma J, Teh BS, Paulino AC. Characteristics and outcome of radiation and chemotherapy-related mucoepidermoid carcinoma of the salivary glands. Pediatr Blood Cancer 2011;57(7):1137–41.

17. Rutt A, Hawkshaw MJ, Lurie D, et al. Salivary gland cancer in patients younger than 30 years. Ear Nose Throat J 2011;90(4):174–84.

18. Ryan JT, El-Naggar AK, Huh W, et al. Primacy of surgery in the management of mucoepidermoid carcinoma in children. Head Neck 2011;33(12):1769–73.

19. Kupferman ME, de la Garza GO, Santillan AA, et al. Outcomes of pediatric patients with malignancies of the major salivary glands. Ann Surg Oncol 2010; 17(12):3301–7.

20. Chiaravalli S, Guzzo M, Bisogno G, et al. Salivary gland carcinomas in children and adolescents; The Italian TREP project experience. Pediatr Blood Cancer 2014;61(11):196–8.

21. Waldron CA, El-Mofty SK, Gnepp DR. Tumors of the intraoral minor salivary glands: a demographic and histologic study of 426 cases. Oral Surg Oral Med Oral Pathol 1988;66:323–33.

22. Dhanuthai K, Boonadulyarat M, Jaengjongdee T, et al. A clinicopathologic study of 311 intra-oral salivary gland tumors in Thais. J Oral Pathol Med 2009; 38:495–500.

23. Galer C, Santillan AA, Chelius D, et al. Minor salivary gland malignancies in the pediatric population. Head Neck 2012;34(11):1648–51.

24. Eversole LR, Rovin S, Sabes WR. Mucoepidermoid carcinoma of minor salivary glands: report of 17 cases with follow-up. J Oral Surg 1972;30(2): 107–12.

25. Olsen KD, Devine KD, Weiland LH. Mucoepidermoid carcinoma of the oral cavity. Otolaryngol Head Neck Surg 1981;89(5):783–91.

26. Conley J, Tinsley PP Jr. Treatment and prognosis of mucoepidermoid carcinoma in the pediatric age group. Arch Otolaryngol 1985;111(5):322–4.

27. Caccamese JF Jr, Ord RA. Paediatric mucoepidermoid carcinoma of the palate. Int J Oral Maxillofac Surg 2002;31(2):136–9.

28. Ord RA, Salama AR. Is it necessary to resect bone for low-grade mucoepidermoid carcinoma of the palate? Br J Oral Maxillofac Surg 2012;50(8):712–4.

29. Bradley P, McClelland L, Mehta D. Pediatric salivary gland epithelial neoplasms. ORL J Otorhinolaryngol Relat Spec 2007;69(3):137–45.

30. Hicks J, Flaitz C. Mucoepidermoid carcinoma of salivary glands in children and adolescents: assessment of proliferation markers. Oral Oncol 2000; 36(5):454–60.

31. Walterhouse DO, Pappo AS, Baker KS, et al. Rhabdomyosarcomas of the parotid region occurring in childhood and adolescence. A report from the Intergroup Rhabdomyosarcoma Study Group. Cancer 2001;92(12):3135–46.

Vascular Malformations and Their Treatment in the Growing Patient

Antonia Kolokythas, DDS, MSc

KEYWORDS

- Vascular anomalies • Vascular tumors • Venous malformations

KEY POINTS

- Vascular anomalies, consistent of vascular tumors and malformations, frequently arise in the head and neck and often occur in the pediatric patient.
- Infantile hemangiomas are the most common tumors in infancy; 10% are found by 1 year of age, with white premature babies and girls affected more often.
- Vascular malformations represent an abnormal proliferation of mature vascular elements, are present at birth, and show equal distribution between the sexes. Vascular malformations grow with the child and are usually affected by hormonal changes with occasional accelerated growth during puberty.
- Capillary-venular and venous malformations represent the most common vascular malformations, approaching 1 in 10,000.
- Lymphangiomas or lymphatic malformations are areas of abnormal development of the lymphatic system of unknown etiology, commonly found in the head and neck region. Surgery, sclerotherapy, and laser treatments have all been used with various success rates in the management of lymphatic malformations.

INTRODUCTION

In 1982, Mulliken and Glowacki proposed a biological classification for these lesions based on their clinical and histologic findings. Based on this classification scheme, which has been supported by subsequent radiographic and biochemical studies, vascular anomalies are classified as hemangiomas (now known as *infantile hemangioma)* and vascular malformations (VMs). This classification was widely adopted and became the official classification of the International Society for the Study of Vascular Anomalies in 1996 with some updates to include infantile hemangioma variants, combined lesions, and other benign vascular origin tumors.[1–7]

Infantile hemangiomas are the most common tumors in infancy, found in as many as 10% of infants by 1 year of age, especially in white and premature babies weighing less than 1000 g, with girls affected 3 to 5 more often than boys. Whites are more prone to hemangioma development, whereas the incidence in African-Americans and Asians is low (1.4% and 0.8%, respectively). Other risk factors include multiparity, advanced maternal age, placental abnormalities (ie, placenta previa). Hemangiomas are proliferative lesions characterized by increased turnover of endothelial cells. Histologic landmarks are the hyperplasia of endothelial cells, which will stain positive for glucose transporter I (in infertile hemangiomas), and the large number of mast cells The lesions appear as

Disclosure Statement: The author has nothing to disclose.

Department of Oral and Maxillofacial Surgery, University of Rochester-Eastman Institute of Oral Health, 625 Elmwood Ave., Rochester, NY 14620, USA

E-mail address: ga1@uic.edu

Oral Maxillofacial Surg Clin N Am 28 (2016) 91–104

http://dx.doi.org/10.1016/j.coms.2015.07.006

solitary lesions in approximately 80% of children, and 60% of the tumors are found in the cervico-facial region. The lesions occur sporadically, although there are some tumors that may follow an autosomal dominant inheritance pattern in familial cases. Hemangiomas may be superficial, deep, or visceral, and, although the location does not alter the biologic behavior, it does affect the clinical manifestations.

The lesions typically appear during the first 2 years of life, if they are not present or evident at birth, as an erythematous patch, telangiectasia, or blanched area when they are located superficially. Deep lesions may appear bluish or a deep purple color, whereas the visceral ones will generally not be evident on clinical examination. Infantile hemangiomas follow a triphasic pattern of evolution during which there is classically a proliferative phase of rapid enlargement that follows and outpaces the child's body growth, which may last for 4 to 8 months before a plateau phase that is consistent with body habitus growth followed by involution. The involution phase starts by age 12 months and usually continues for the next 5 to 7 years. Roughly half of the lesions involute by age 5, and 70% by 7 years of age, but the process may continue until adolescence. Even with complete involution, some clinical signs of the tumor may still be evident on physical examination.[8–16]

VMs, represent an abnormal proliferation of mature vascular elements, are present at birth, and show equal distribution between the sexes. The lesion grows with the child and is usually affected by hormonal changes with occasional accelerated growth during puberty. Unlike hemangiomas, histopathologically there is no proliferation of endothelial cells, and the number of mast cells is normal. The lesions tend to infiltrate surrounding normal tissues, which makes their management challenging.

Further subclassification of VMs is based either on the type of vessels involved (capillary, venous, arterial, lymphatic, or combined forms) or the flow characteristics of the lesion (low- vs high-flow VMs). High-flow VMs are arteriovenous malformations (AVMs), whereas low-flow lesions are capillary-venular malformations or venous or lymphatic malformations (LMs). VMs are present at birth, as they represent errors in morphogenesis but, unlike hemangiomas, may go undetected until later in life, even into the teenage years; they do not regress and continue to expand with time.

The clinical appearance and characteristics vary according to the type of VM lesion. A palpable thrill or audible bruit, for example, may be evident in high-flow lesions, whereas diascopy can help distinguish venous malformations from subcutaneous or deep hemangiomas, as both may appear bluish or clinical examination. Diascopy is performed by pressing a glass slide over the lesion and observing for blanching of the bluish/deep purple color as blood is evacuated from the VM; whereas, in contrast, no color change is noted when diascopy is performed on a hemangioma.

HIGH-FLOW LESIONS
Arteriovenous Malformations

AVMs of the head and neck are among the most aggressive of VMs that often cause significant deformities and functional limitations. Although the exact etiology and pathogenesis of AVMs are currently unknown, defects of the transforming growth factor-beta signaling and a genetic 2-hit hypothesis seem to be the 2 most likely candidate theories. Although most of these lesions are present at birth, they are often misdiagnosed as other vascular lesions, or they lack classic presentation for appropriate diagnosis. Often cases are described as appearing in adults after trauma, or a rapid expansion is noted during puberty. Regardless of presentation, these lesions are characterized by direct connections between the arterial and venous system without intervening capillaries.[8,13,14,17–19]

Seventy percent of the AVMs in the head and neck involve the midface, with the cheek, nose, and forehead the most commonly involved sites. AVMs can invade the underlying tissues and the bone of the midface or the mandible, causing significant destruction and further complicating treatment. Interestingly, some of the intraosseous lesions diagnosed as hemangiomas do represent VMs (usually low flow) based on histologic examination and immunostaining. AVMs are staged based on presentation and clinical examination. Stage I AVMs are the quiescent lesions with only minimal clinical findings; stage II lesions show expansion, palpable thrills, or bruits or pulsations; stage III lesions are those that invade adjacent structures causing destruction, pain, ulceration, or bleeding; stage IV lesions cause congestive heart failure owing to decompensation from the rapid uncontrolled growth.[13,17,20,21]

Diagnosis of Arteriovenous Malformations

Clinical examination and imaging are crucial in the diagnosis of AVMs. Imaging, either contrast-enhanced computed tomography (CT) or MRI will distinguish between VMs and vascular tumors. The VM will lack a discrete soft tissue mass and will have enlarged feeding and draining vessels. Areas of thrombosis or intralesional hemorrhage may be found within the VM as well. Magnetic esonance angiogram and/or CT angiogram are essential for evaluation of the flow dynamics, examination of the detailed vascular anatomy, determination of extent of the lesion, and treatment planning. Classically, one or most commonly multiple hypertrophied arterial feeders will be identified shunting rapidly into the enlarged draining venous system across a nidus without a normal intervening capillary network.[8,13,20,22–24]

Management of Arteriovenous Malformations

Management of AVMs consists of surgical extirpation, embolization alone, and embolization followed by surgical resection. The extent of the lesion and involvement of adjacent vital structures make treatment of head and neck AVMs, especially in the growing patient, challenging. The watchful waiting approach, for lesions in children without expansion or obvious deformities, used in the past, is falling out of favor because of the known challenges associated with rapid growth during adolescence and persistence of the disease process. Intravascular embolization alone provides temporary control of the AVM, but because of the extremely high recurrence rate, worsening of symptoms is reserved today for control of active bleeding, ulcerations, or incurable cases. The reason for the high recurrence rate after monotherapy with embolization is thought to be the recruitment of new vessels and collateralization for support portions of the nidus that have gone undetected. Often serial embolizations are required especially for extensive lesions.[8,13,16,25,26]

Small, very localized lesions can be surgically removed with good long-term outcomes. Ideally preoperative supraselective embolization, followed by meticulous tissue removal and appropriate reconstruction, is the treatment of choice and can provide high cure rates for small lesions. Unfortunately, even with this dual modality treatment, recurrence rates for diffuse AVMs are still unacceptably

high (>90%). Excision is undertaken 24 to 48 hours after embolization to allow for better control of blood loss and better definition of the surgical margins. Extreme care should be exercised during embolization to occlude the nidus only or the arteriovenous shunts and avoid the normal vasculature. Absolute ethanol, cyanoacrylate glue, or Onyx (an ethylene-vinyl alcohol copolymer) are the various agents used for embolization of AVMs. Despite the local and perivascular inflammation caused by Onyx and the tattooing of the overlying skin (because of the dimethyl-sulfoxide), it appears to have gained popularity for treatment of both extracranial and intracranial AVMs.[27] Specific sites such as the ear or tip of the nose, mandible, or maxilla may require specific techniques and should be individualized.[8,13,14,19,21,25,26,28,29]

Figs. 1–14 document 2 cases of intraosseous AVMs, the radiographic presentation, treatment rendered, and outcomes over 5 years.

LOW-FLOW LESIONS
Capillary-Venular Malformations/Venous Malformations

Capillary-venular and venous malformations are discussed together (using one term, *low-flow vascular malformations* [LFVMs]), as their distinction is solely based on clinical and ultrasound examination findings, and their presentation and treatment do not differ significantly (**Figs. 15** and **16**). LFVMs represent the most common VMs with an incident approaching 1 in 10,000. They comprise various size venous channels and present as soft comprisable lesions, often in a segmental fashion, which are usually present at birth. The congestion, thrombosis of the various venous connections, and the elasticity of the vessels over time cause expansion of the lesion, formation of phleboliths (calcified thrombi), and even pain that make treatment necessary. Venous malformations do not regress. Although most LFVMs appear sporadically, cases associated

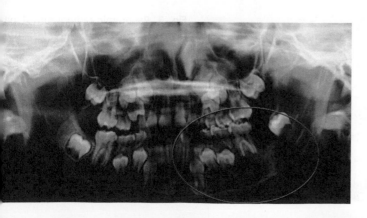

Fig. 1. Panoramic radiograph of a 10-year-old girl with a stage I AVM involving the left posterior mandible. *Circle* indicate lesions.

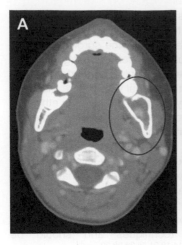
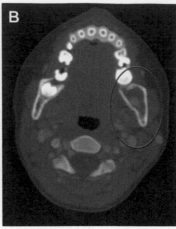

Fig. 2. Axial CT scan with contrast soft tissue (*A*), and bony (*B*) window showing an intrabony nonhomogeneous mass of the left posterior mandible. *Circle* indicate lesions.

with autosomal dominant inheritance pattern have been identified. In multiple sporadic and solitary lesions, a loss of function mutation on the angiopoietin receptor gene TIE2/TEK has been identified as has been upregulation of several growth factors, including transforming growth factor-β and β-fibroblast growth factor. Growth of LFVMs associated with hormonal changes such as during puberty and pregnancy is at least in part explained by the presence of progesterone receptors. For the group of lesions that are not thought to be sporadic, the genetic locus is identified in chromosome 9p. Finally, elevated D-dimers is recently identified as a disease biomarker and can be associated with localized intravascular coagulopathy, putting the patient at risk for disseminated intravascular coagulopathy during treatment.[8,13,14,30–36]

Venus malformations can be localized or diffuse and superficial or deep, and the latter dictates the surface color characteristics and are often found in the head neck. For example, deeply located lesions cause no discoloration of the overlying skin or mucosa but may cause visible swelling and protrusion, whereas superficial ones with skin or mucosal involvement are responsible for the deep blue or purple color. Characteristically LFVMs will swell with hydrostatic pressure changes, such as when the involved body part is dependent, or with maneuvers that prevent venous return, such as Valsalva or squatting. Symptoms are directly related to the location of the lesions and they can either be completely asymptomatic, perhaps only a cosmetic concern, or cause visual, respiratory, or speech and mastication issues. Lesions involving the airway or in proximity to the airway may cause symptoms of sleep apnea and, along with those involving or in proximity to the eyes, pose significant treatment challenges.[37–40]

Diagnosis of Venous Malformations

The clinical presentation outlined above combined with imaging in the form of ultrasound scan (US), CT, or MRI will help establish the diagnosis

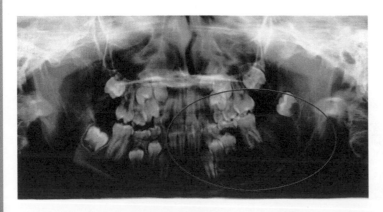

Fig. 3. Panoramic radiograph of patient 6 months after initial presentation now with stage II AVM involving the left posterior mandible. *Circle* indicate lesions.

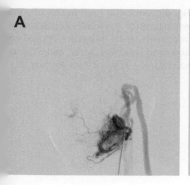
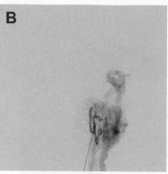

Fig. 4. Diagnostic angiogram shows the left mandibular AVM with feeder vessels from both the facial (*A*) and lingual (*B*) arteries.

distinguish between the variants, and evaluate the extent of the lesion. There is no role for angiography for diagnostic purposes, but it can be used for treatment purposes or for evaluation for presence of mixed lesions. On US, LFVMs will be of mixed echogenicity, compressible, purely monophasic, or with no flow. The presence of biphasic flow indicates a mixed lesion, usually a capillary-venular malformation. MRI will easily identify the extent of the lesion, involvement of vital structures, and extension into surrounding tissues while avoiding unnecessary radiation exposure to the growing patient. LFVMs showed contrast enhancement, which helps with differentiation from other malformations that in the head and neck include lymphangiomas and cystic hygromas, thyroglossal duct cysts, and branchial cleft cysts that are all nonenhancing on MRI (**Figs. 17** and **18**).[24,41–44]

Treatment of Venous Malformations

Percutaneous sclerotherapy and neodymium-doped yttrium aluminum garnet laser therapy have emerged as the most preferred treatment options for venous malformations. Surgical resection can be also be used and perhaps has a role for small, well-localized lesions (See **Fig. 15**). Often, multimodality therapy is indicated for extensive lesions, especially those involving vital structures and the airway. Several sclerosing agents, such as ethanol, 3% sodium tetradecyl sulfate, and bleomycin have been used successfully in the treatment of these lesions with or without imaging guidance. Ethanol is the most potent and perhaps the most successful agent in minimizing recurrences and yet the one associated with the most severe complications. Issues with ethanol injections include damage to overlying skin or mucosa when involved by the lesion, risk of extravasation into surrounding structures causing damage, and neurologic injury. Low doses not exceeding 1 mg/kg and administration in increments of 0.1 mL/kg every 5 minutes are key to decreasing the risk of cardiovascular collapse. The recent formulations with imported viscosity of ethanol preparations, ethanol gel, and ethylcellulose-ethanol have improved ethanol's safety as sclerosing agent for LFVMs. Bleomycin A5 made a return in 2010 after Hou and colleagues[45] reported successful

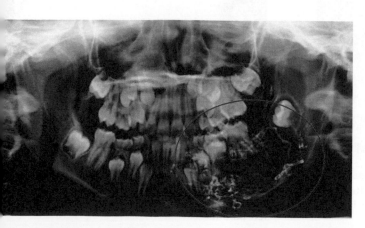

Fig. 5. Panoramic radiograph of left posterior mandible stage II AVM after embolization with Onyx. *Circle* indicate lesions.

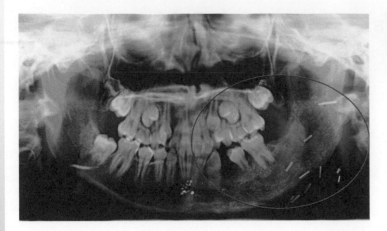

Fig. 6. Panoramic radiograph of AVM left posterior mandible 2 years after treatment with selective embolization and excision after removal of hardware. *Circle* indicate lesions.

treatment of venous malformations in the cervico-facial region in Chinese patients. Because of the high risk for pulmonary and renal failure with use of bleomycin, close monitoring of these patients for both pulmonary and renal function should be undertaken. Close monitoring after sclerotherapy is mandatory, especially for lesions involving or close to the airway and the tongue because of the significant soft edema that occurs several hours after treatment (see **Fig. 18**; **Figs. 19** and **20**). Consideration should be given to keeping the patient intubated overnight or at least under close observation after treatment for monitoring of airway compromise.[46–57]

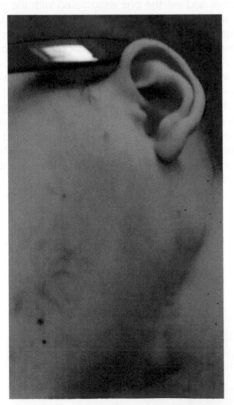

Fig. 7. Facial skin appearance 3 years after treatment, selective embolization and excision of left posterior mandible AVM. Note discoloration.

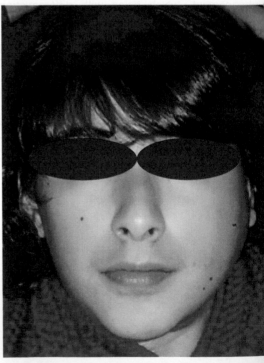

Fig. 8. Patient 6 years after diagnosis and treatment of left posterior mandible AVM, with new-onset facial swelling from recurrence of AVM with involvement of left parotid.

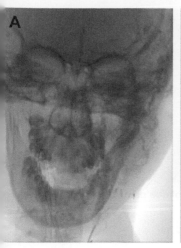
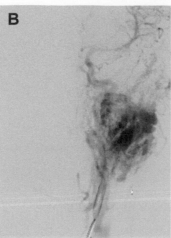

Fig. 9. Diagnostic angiogram shows left face AVM recurrence with no bone involvement but with extensive involvement of the left parotid gland. (*A*) Anteroposterior plane skull film. (*B*) Representative view of the AVM during angiography.

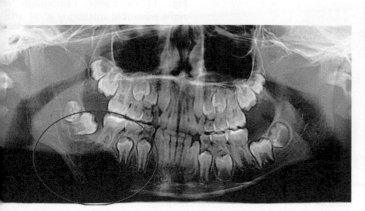

Fig. 10. Panoramic radiograph of 12-year-old girl with stage II AVM involving the right posterior mandible. *Circle* indicate lesions.

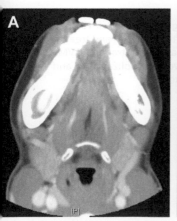
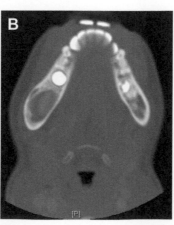

Fig. 11. Axial CT scan with contrast. Soft tissue (*A*) and bony (*B*) windows show an intrabony nonhomogeneous mass of the right posterior mandible.

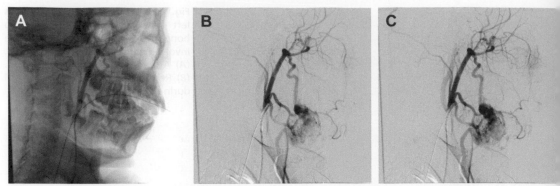

Fig. 12. Diagnostic angiogram shows right mandible intrabony AVM. (*A*) Oblique plane skull film. (*B*, *C*) Repre sentative view of the AVM during angiography shows progressive fill.

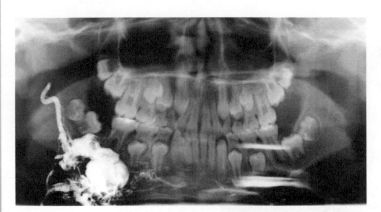

Fig. 13. Panoramic radiograph o right mandible intrabony AVM after selective embolization.

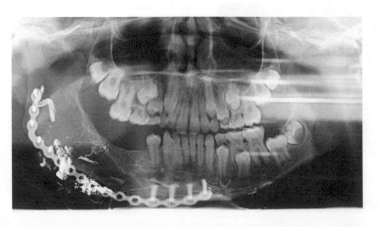

Fig. 14. Panoramic radiograph 5 year after diagnosis and treatment of right mandible intrabony AVM with selec tive embolization and surgica excision.

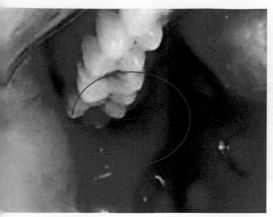

Fig. 15. Localized venous malformation right posterior palate adjacent to #1. *Circle* indicate lesions.

Capillary Malformations

Facial capillary malformations are most often associated with Sturge-Weber syndrome and are described as port wine stains. Classically, they present on the skin of the face in the distribution of cranial nerve V, often with involvement of the leptomeninges and associated neurologic complications. Ipsilateral ocular, nasal, and oral cavity involvement are characteristic of the capillary malformations associated with Sturge-Weber syndrome. Lesions can cause significant facial disfigurement, owing to thickening and nodularity, and seizures, developmental delay, and migraines owing the intracranial extension. Therapy with pulsed dye laser is the recommended treatment for capillary malformations, whereas appropriate workup and symptom-oriented treatment should be undertaken for patients with Sturge-Weber syndrome.[14,58,59] Isolated lesions, although less common, often involve the oral cavity.

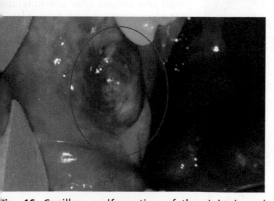

Fig. 16. Capillary malformation of the right buccal mucosa. *Circle* indicate lesions.

Lymphatic Malformations

Lymphangiomas or lymphatic malformations (LM) are areas of abnormal development of the lymphatic system of unknown etiology, commonly found in the head and neck region (70% of the cases). Approximately 50% of the lesions are present at birth most, approximately 90%, are identified by the age of 2 years. The incidence of LM is reported between 1.2% and 2.8% with equal gender distribution. Two types of LM are described: macrocystic and microcystic. Additionally, LMs can be described based on the fluid contents of the cystic spaces, either as serous or chylous. Histologically, cystic spaces most appropriately termed *sacs* or *dilated locules* are identified. These are lined by endothelium supported by connective tissue stroma with scattered lymphocyte follicle cells and occasionally germinal centers. Staging of LMs is based on location and extent of the lesion: stage I, unilateral infrahyoid; stage II, unilateral suprahyoid; stage III, unilateral infrasuprahyoid; and stage IV, bilateral infrasuprahyoid. Spontaneous regression of the lesion, although reported, is rare and usually followed by recurrence in long-term follow-up. In general, LMs of the neck tend to be macrocystic and well demarcated with somewhat clear separation from the surrounding tissues, whereas those in the oral cavity and tongue are more often microcytic and ill defined.[60–64]

Diagnosis of Lymphatic Malformations

Superficially located (mucosal or skin) LMs typically present as small yellow fluid-filled vesicles. More deeply situated lesions may cause hypertrophy or macrosomia and significant disfigurement. Symptoms are closely associated with the location and extent of the LM and are key to diagnosis along with clinical examination and imaging. Rapid enlargement or size alterations are classically noted with recent infections (commonly upper respiratory infections) or trauma or caused by bleeding within the LM. As slow flow-lesions they will appear as nonenhancing, intermediate signal intensity lesions on MRI. Both US and MRI are equally appropriate imaging modalities for diagnosis of LMs, with the expected superiority of MRI in evaluation of the exact extent and involvement of the lesion.[3,8,13,60,65–68]

Treatment of Lymphatic Malformations

Treatment of LMs is based on several factors that include symptomatology, anatomic location, onset of presentation, and growth rate among others. It is important to individualize treatment with a

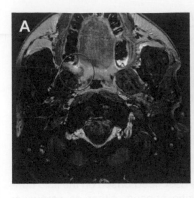

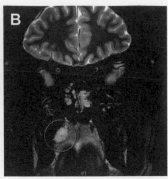

Fig. 17. (A) Axial cut, T2 MRI of the face shows a hyperintense ovoid soft tissue lesion measuring 1.5 × 1.1 × 1.8 cm within the right soft palate posterior to #1 right maxillary molar. On contrast administration, this lesion shows peripheral nodular appearing incomplete. Diagnosis: Venous malformation enhancement. (B) Coronal cut T2 MRI image of the face shows the hyperintense lesion on the right posterior hard palate. Diagnosis: Venous malformation. *Circle* indicate lesions.

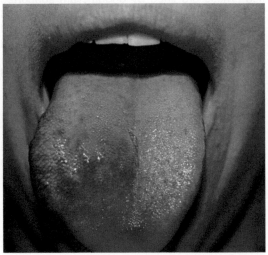

Fig. 18. Venous malformation involving the right oral tongue.

multidisciplinary team approach. The possibility of severe disfigurement for extensive lesions of the head and neck should be carefully considered when deciding the best treatment modality. An elegant detailed discussion of treatment guidelines for head and neck LMs was published by Zhou and colleagues[60] in 2011. The key treatment modalities are discussed here. Surgery, sclerotherapy, and laser treatments have all been used with various success rates in the management of LMs.[69–71]

Among numerous agents used over the years, such as doxycycline, hypertonic glucose solution and ethanol, bleomycin A5 and OK-432 are the mainstay therapy. Specifically, Pingyangmycin (a single-component A5), because of its overall safety, low cost, and availability, is the agent used as single-modality therapy or in combination with surgical resection. According to Perkins and colleagues[66] the most important aspect of the technique for high success rates is removal of the fluid from within the LM. Fever, malaise, and skin rash are not uncommon, whereas severe

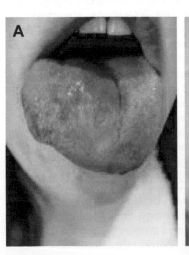

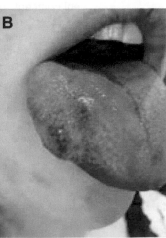

Fig. 19. Venous malformation of the right oral tongue after sclerotherapy (A) immediately and (B) 1 hour later. Patient had no pain or discomfort.

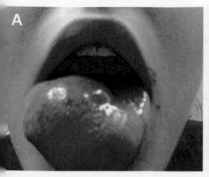
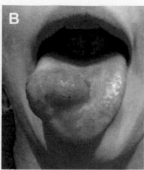

Fig. 20. Venous malformation of the right oral tongue after sclerotherapy (A) 8 hours after injection and (B) 12 hours after injection. Patient had no pain or discomfort.

allergic reactions that can be threatening are less common but a possibility. Patients require close observation for signs of allergic reaction that requires immediate attention.[72–76]

OK-432, or picibanil, is a lyophilized powder containing cells of *Streptococcus pyogenes Su* strain that is treated with benzyl penicillin. A skin test to ensure there is no allergy to penicillin is mandatory before treatment with OK-432. The agent causes obliteration of the lymphatic channels due to stimulation of lymphatic endothelial cells, with only minimal fibrosis. Obviously both agents can only be used in macrocytic lesions, as they require deposition within the cystic spaces.[60,77,78]

Carbon dioxide, neodymium-doped yttrium aluminum garnet laser can be used to successfully treat superficial lesions especially when infected. Bleeding control and minimal or no pain with ability for multiple treatments are the major benefits of the use of lasers for management of LMs. Combination therapy with CO_2 laser and sclerosing agent can be successful in management of superficial lesions in the oral cavity. Alternatively, surgical resection of localized hyperplastic lesions can be followed by laser treatment of any residual disease or sclerosing therapy.[79,80]

Surgical resection of macrocystic LMs in the head and neck is less challenging, as these are usually well defined and can be safely and adequately removed. Microcystic lesions, on the other hand, can be extremely challenging to resect because of ill-defined borders and intimate involvement of vital structures. Lesions that are not life threatening can be addressed later in life, avoiding disfigurement and growth alterations in the pediatric patient. Appropriate reconstruction to restore form and function should be planned when surgery is required for removal of aggressive disfiguring lesions.[81–85]

Summary

VMs and vascular tumors of the head and neck in the growing patient are challenging to treat and often disfiguring. Early diagnosis and intervention at appropriate time based on the patient age and the lesion behavior are keys to successful outcomes. A multidisciplinary team consisting of pediatric specialists including interventional radiology/neuroradiology, oral and maxillofacial surgery, otolaryngology, and plastic and reconstructive surgery is needed for the treatment of these patients. Long-term follow-up is required because of the high recurrence rates of these lesions.

REFERENCES

1. Glowacki J, Mulliken JB. Mast cells in hemangiomas and vascular malformations. Pediatrics 1982;70(1): 48–51.
2. Mulliken JB, Glowacki J. Classification of pediatric vascular lesions. Plast Reconstr Surg 1982;70(1): 120–1.
3. Mulliken JB, Glowacki J. Hemangiomas and vascular malformations in infants and children: a classification based on endothelial characteristics. Plast Reconstr Surg 1982;69(3):412–22.
4. Garzon MCH, Huang JT, Enjolras O, et al. Vascular malformations. Part II: associated syndromes. J Am Acad Dermatol 2007;56(4):541–64.
5. Garzon MC, Huang JT, Enjolras O, et al. Vascular malformations: Part I. J Am Acad Dermatol 2007; 56(3):353–70 [quiz: 371–4].
6. Enjolras O. Classification and management of the various superficial vascular anomalies: hemangiomas and vascular malformations. J Dermatol 1997;24(11):701–10.
7. Enjolras OM, Mulliken JB. Vascular tumors and vascular malformations (new issues). Adv Dermatol 1997;13:375–423.
8. Richter GT, Friedman AB. Hemangiomas and vascular malformations: current theory and management. Int J Pediatr 2012;2012:645678.
9. Chamlin SLH, Haggstrom AN, Drolet BA, et al. Multicenter prospective study of ulcerated hemangiomas. J Pediatr 2007;151(6):684–9, 689.e1.

10. Haggstrom AND, Drolet BA, Baselga E, et al. Prospective study of infantile hemangiomas: demographic, prenatal, and perinatal characteristics. J Pediatr 2007;150(3):291–4.

11. Jacobs AH, Walton RG. The incidence of birthmarks in the neonate. Pediatrics 1976;58(2):218–22.

12. Amir J, Metzker A, Krikler R, et al. Strawberry hemangioma in preterm infants. Pediatr Dermatol 1986; 3(4):331–2.

13. Puttgen KBP, Pearl M, Tekes A, et al. Update on pediatric extracranial vascular anomalies of the head and neck. Childs Nerv Syst 2010;26(10):1417–33.

14. Eivazi B, Werner JA. Management of vascular malformations and hemangiomas of the head and neck–an update. Curr Opin Otolaryngol Head Neck Surg 2013;21(2):157–63.

15. Marler JJ, Mulliken JB. Current management of hemangiomas and vascular malformations. Clin Plast Surg 2005;32(1):99–116, ix.

16. Eivazi BW, Wiegand S, Negm H, et al. Orbital and periorbital vascular anomalies–an approach to diagnosis and therapeutic concepts. Acta Otolaryngol 2010;130(8):942–51.

17. Kohout MP, Hansen M, Pribaz JJ, et al. Arteriovenous malformations of the head and neck: natural history and management. Plast Reconstr Surg 1998;102(3):643–54.

18. Buckmiller LMR, Richter GT, Suen JY. Diagnosis and management of hemangiomas and vascular malformations of the head and neck. Oral Dis 2010;16(5): 405–18.

19. Richter GTS, Suen JY. Clinical course of arteriovenous malformations of the head and neck: a case series. Otolaryngol Head Neck Surg 2010;142(2):184–90.

20. Burrows PE, Mulliken JB, Fellows KE, et al. Childhood hemangiomas and vascular malformations: angiographic differentiation. AJR Am J Roentgenol 1983;141(3):483–8.

21. Bradley JP, Zide BM, Berenstein A, et al. Large arteriovenous malformations of the face: aesthetic results with recurrence control. Plast Reconstr Surg 1999;103(2):351–61.

22. Burrows PE, Laor T, Paltiel H, et al. Diagnostic imaging in the evaluation of vascular birthmarks. Dermatol Clin 1998;16(3):455–88.

23. Tao Q, LV B, Bhatia KS, et al. Three-dimensional CT angiography for the diagnosis and assessment of arteriovenous malformations in the oral and maxillofacial region. J Craniomaxillofac Surg 2009;38(1): 32–7.

24. Konez O, Burrows PE. Magnetic resonance of vascular anomalies. Magn Reson Imaging Clin N Am 2002;10(2):363–88, vii.

25. Fearon JA. Discussion. Extracranial arteriovenous malformations: natural progression and recurrence after treatment. Plast Reconstr Surg 2010;125(4): 1195–6.

26. Richter GTS, Suen J, North PE, et al. Arteriovenous malformations of the tongue: a spectrum of disease. Laryngoscope 2007;117(2):328–35.

27. Thiex R, Wu I, Mulliken JB, et al. Safety and clinical efficacy of Onyx for embolization of extracranial head and neck vascular anomalies. AJNR Am J Neuroradiol 2011;32(6):1082–6.

28. Visser AF, FitzJohn T, Tan ST. Surgical management of arteriovenous malformation. J Plast Reconstr Aesthet Surg 2010;64(3):283–91.

29. Arat A, Cil BE, Vargel I, et al. Embolization of high-flow craniofacial vascular malformations with onyx. AJNR Am J Neuroradiol 2007;28(7):1409–14.

30. Dubova EA, Podgornova MN, Schegolev AI. Expression of adhesion molecules and cyclin d1 in cells of solid-pseudopapillary tumors of the pancreas. Bull Exp Biol Med 2009;148(6):908–10.

31. Pavlov KA, Dubova EA, Shchyogolev AI, et al. Expression of growth factors in endotheliocytes in vascular malformations. Bull Exp Biol Med 2009; 147(3):366–70.

32. Boon LM, Mulliken JB, Vikkula M, et al. Assignment of a locus for dominantly inherited venous malformations to chromosome 9p. Hum Mol Genet 1994;3(9): 1583–7.

33. Limaye N, Boon LM, Vikkula M. From germline towards somatic mutations in the pathophysiology of vascular anomalies. Hum Mol Genet 2009;18(R1): R65–74.

34. Limaye N, Wouters V, Uebelhoer M, et al. Somatic mutations in angiopoietin receptor gene TEK cause solitary and multiple sporadic venous malformations. Nat Genet 2009;41(1):118–24.

35. Duyka LJ, Fan CY, Coviello-Malle JM, et al. Progesterone receptors identified in vascular malformations of the head and neck. Otolaryngol Head Neck Surg 2009;141(4):491–5.

36. Wouters VL, Limaye N, Uebelhoer M, et al. Hereditary cutaneomucosal venous malformations are caused by TIE2 mutations with widely variable hyper-phosphorylating effects. Eur J Hum Genet 2009;18(4):414–20.

37. Boon LM, Mulliken JB, Enjolras O, et al. Glomuvenous malformation (glomangioma) and venous malformation: distinct clinicopathologic and genetic entities. Arch Dermatol 2004;140(8):971–6.

38. Dompmartin A, Vikkula M, Boon LM. Venous malformation: update on aetiopathogenesis, diagnosis and management. Phlebology 2010;25(5):224–35.

39. Ohlms LA, Forsen J, Burrows PE. Venous malformation of the pediatric airway. Int J Pediatr Otorhinolaryngol 1996;37(2):99–114.

40. Glade RS, Richter GT, James CA, et al. Diagnosis and management of pediatric cervicofacial venous malformations: retrospective review from a vascular anomalies center. Laryngoscope 2009; 120(2):229–35.

41. Trop I, Dubois J, Guibaud L, et al. Soft-tissue venous malformations in pediatric and young adult patients: diagnosis with Doppler US. Radiology 1999;212(3): 841–5.

42. Gelbert F, Riche MC, Reizine D, et al. MR imaging of head and neck vascular malformations. J Magn Reson Imaging 1991;1(5):579–84.

43. Mourier KL, Gelbert F, Assouline E, et al. MRI in multiple vascular lesions: identification of the ruptured malformation. Acta Neurochir (Wien) 1991;112(3–4):83–7.

44. Robertson RL, Robson CD, Barnes PD, et al. Head and neck vascular anomalies of childhood. Neuroimaging Clin N Am 1999;9(1):115–32.

45. Hou R, Guo J, Hu K, et al. A clinical study of ultrasound -guided intralesional injection of bleomycin A5 on venous malformation in cervical-facial region in China. J Vasc Surg 2010;51:940–5.

46. Wong GA, Armstrong DC, Robertson JM. Cardiovascular collapse during ethanol sclerotherapy in a pediatric patient. Paediatr Anaesth 2006;16(3):343–6.

47. Lacey B, Rootman J, Marotta TR. Distensible venous malformations of the orbit: clinical and hemodynamic features and a new technique of management. Ophthalmology 1999;106(6):1197–209.

48. Glade R, Vinson K, Richter G, et al. Endoscopic management of airway venous malformations with Nd:YAG laser. Ann Otol Rhinol Laryngol 2010; 119(5):289–93.

49. Kang GC, Song C. Forty-one cervicofacial vascular anomalies and their surgical treatment–retrospection and review. Ann Acad Med Singapore 2008; 37(3):165–79.

50. Choi DJ, Alomari AI, Chaudry G, et al. Neurointerventional management of low-flow vascular malformations of the head and neck. Neuroimaging Clin N Am 2009;19(2):199–218.

51. Lee CH, Chen SG. Direct percutaneous ethanol instillation for treatment of venous malformation in the face and neck. Br J Plast Surg 2005;58(8): 1073–8.

52. Tan ST, Bialostocki A, Brasch H, et al. Venous malformation of the orbit. J Oral Maxillofac Surg 2004; 62(10):1308–11.

53. Diolaiuti S, Iizuka T, Schroth G, et al. Orbital venous malformation: percutaneous treatment using an electrolytically detachable fibred coil. Acta Ophthalmol 2009;87(2):229–32.

54. Kishimoto Y, Hirano S, Kato N, et al. Endoscopic KTP laser photocoagulation therapy for pharyngolaryngeal venous malformations in adults. Ann Otol Rhinol Laryngol 2008;117(12):881–5.

55. Andreisek G, Nanz D, Weishaupt D, et al. MR imaging-guided percutaneous sclerotherapy of peripheral venous malformations with a clinical 1.5-T unit: a pilot study. J Vasc Interv Radiol 2009;20(7): 879–87.

56. Mitchell SE, Shah AM, Schwengel D. Pulmonary artery pressure changes during ethanol embolization procedures to treat vascular malformations: can cardiovascular collapse be predicted? J Vasc Interv Radiol 2006;17(2 Pt 1):253–62.

57. Berenguer B, Burrows PE, Zurakowski D, et al. Sclerotherapy of craniofacial venous malformations: complications and results. Plast Reconstr Surg 1999;104(1):1–11 [discussion: 12–5].

58. Eivazi B, Roessler M, Pfützner W, et al. Port-wine stains are more than skin-deep! Expanding the spectrum of extracutaneous manifestations of nevi flammei of the head and neck. Eur J Dermatol 2012;22(2):246–51.

59. Faurschou A, Olesen AB, Leonardi-Bee J, et al. Lasers or light sources for treating port-wine stains. Cochrane Database Syst Rev 2011;(11):CD007152.

60. Zhou Q, Zheng JW, Mai HM, et al. Treatment guidelines of lymphatic malformations of the head and neck. Oral Oncol 2011;47(12):1105–9.

61. Kennedy TL. Cystic hygroma-lymphangioma: a rare and still unclear entity. Laryngoscope 1989;99(10 Pt 2 Suppl 49):1–10.

62. Hancock BJ, St-Vil D, Luks FI, et al. Complications of lymphangiomas in children. J Pediatr Surg 1992; 27(2):220–4 [discussion: 224–6].

63. de Serres LM, Sie KC, Richardson MA. Lymphatic malformations of the head and neck. A proposal for staging. Arch Otolaryngol Head Neck Surg 1995;121(5):577–82.

64. Boyd JB, Mulliken JB, Kaban LB, et al. Skeletal changes associated with vascular malformations. Plast Reconstr Surg 1984;74(6):789–97.

65. Arnold R, Chaudry G. Diagnostic imaging of vascular anomalies. Clin Plast Surg 2010;38(1): 21–9.

66. Perkins JA, Manning SC, Tempero RM, et al. Lymphatic malformations: review of current treatment. Otolaryngol Head Neck Surg 2010;142(6): 795–803, 803.e1.

67. Perkins JA, Manning SC, Tempero RM, et al. Lymphatic malformations: current cellular and clinical investigations. Otolaryngol Head Neck Surg 2010;142(6):789–94.

68. Perkins JA, Maniglia C, Magit A, et al. Clinical and radiographic findings in children with spontaneous lymphatic malformation regression. Otolaryngol Head Neck Surg 2008;138(6):772–7.

69. Dubois J, Garel L, Abela A, et al. Lymphangiomas in children: percutaneous sclerotherapy with an alcoholic solution of zein. Radiology 1997;204(3):651–4.

70. Burrows PE, Mitri RK, Alomari A, et al. Percutaneous sclerotherapy of lymphatic malformations with doxycycline. Lymphat Res Biol 2008;6(3–4):209–16.

71. Bai Y, Jia J, Huang XX, et al. Sclerotherapy of microcystic lymphatic malformations in oral and facial regions. J Oral Maxillofac Surg 2009;67(2):251–6.

72. Yura J, Hashimoto T, Tsuruga N, et al. Bleomycin treatment for cystic hygroma in children. Nihon Geka Hokan 1977;46(5):607–14.

73. Bloom DC, Perkins JA, Manning SC. Management of lymphatic malformations. Curr Opin Otolaryngol Head Neck Surg 2004;12(6):500–4.

74. Sainsbury DC, Kessell G, Fall AJ, et al. Intralesional bleomycin injection treatment for vascular birthmarks: a 5-year experience at a single United Kingdom unit. Plast Reconstr Surg 2011;127(5):2031–44.

75. Zheng JW, Yang XJ, Wang YA, et al. Intralesional injection of Pingyangmycin for vascular malformations in oral and maxillofacial regions: an evaluation of 297 consecutive patients. Oral Oncol 2009;45(10): 872–6.

76. Zhong PQ, Zhi FX, Li R, et al. Long-term results of intratumorous bleomycin-A5 injection for head and neck lymphangioma. Oral Surg Oral Med Oral Pathol Oral Radiol Endod 1998;86(2):139–44.

77. Smith MC, Zimmerman MB, Burke DK, et al. Efficacy and safety of OK-432 immunotherapy of lymphatic malformations. Laryngoscope 2009;119(1):107–15.

78. Ogita S, Tsuto T, Nakamura K, et al. OK-432 therapy for lymphangioma in children: why and how does it work? J Pediatr Surg 1996;31(4):477–80.

79. Glade RS, Buckmiller LM. CO2 laser resurfacing of intraoral lymphatic malformations: a 10-year experience. Int J Pediatr Otorhinolaryngol 2009; 73(10):1358–61.

80. Angiero F, Benedicenti S, Benedicenti A, et al. Head and neck hemangiomas in pediatric patients treated with endolesional 980-nm diode laser. Photomed Laser Surg 2009;27(4):553–9.

81. Boardman SJ, Cochrane LA, Roebuck D, et al. Multimodality treatment of pediatric lymphatic malformations of the head and neck using surgery and sclerotherapy. Arch Otolaryngol Head Neck Surg 2010;136(3):270–6.

82. Zeng RS, Liu XQ, Wang AX, et al. Sequential treatment of giant lymphatic malformation of the tongue combined with severe oral and maxillofacial deformities. J Oral Maxillofac Surg 2008;66(11):2364–71.

83. Greene AK, Burrows PE, Smith L, et al. Periorbital lymphatic malformation: clinical course and management in 42 patients. Plast Reconstr Surg 2005; 115(1):22–30.

84. Padwa BL, Hayward PG, Ferraro NF, et al. Cervicofacial lymphatic malformation: clinical course, surgical intervention, and pathogenesis of skeletal hypertrophy. Plast Reconstr Surg 1995;95(6):951–60.

85. Edwards PD, Rahbar R, Ferraro NF, et al. Lymphatic malformation of the lingual base and oral floor. Plast Reconstr Surg 2005;115(7):1906–15.

Pediatric Vascular Tumors of the Head and Neck

Carl Bouchard, DMD, MSc, FRCD(C)[a],*, Zachary S. Peacock, DMD, MD[b],
Maria J. Troulis, DDS, MSc[c]

KEYWORDS

• Hemangiomas • Vascular • Lesions • Pediatric

KEY POINTS

• There is confusion regarding the classification of vascular neoplasms and malformations of the head and neck.
• An incorrect diagnosis of hemangioma is often posed.
• The diagnosis of a vascular tumor is mostly based on history and physical examination.
• Giant cell lesions, pyogenic granulomas, and aneurysmal bone cysts are not vascular neoplasms per se, but they have a prominent vascular component.
• Other rare pediatric vascular lesions include hemangioendothelioma, tufted angioma, and juvenile nasopharyngeal angiofibroma.

INTRODUCTION

Vascular tumors of the head and neck are commonly seen in the pediatric population. Oral and maxillofacial surgeons are often involved in the treatment of these children, particularly if there is bony involvement, or an association with the dentition. The diagnosis and treatment of vascular tumors, particularly those of the head and neck, have been hampered by a confusing nomenclature. An incorrect diagnosis of hemangioma is often posed, even in the presence of lesions that do not regress.

Mulliken and Glowacki[1] suggested a simplified classification based on endothelial characteristics. Vascular lesions are divided into 2 categories: vascular tumors and malformations. Hemangiomas are tumors of endothelial cells, whereas vascular malformations are the result of a structural anomaly of the blood vessels with normal endothelial cells. A detailed classification, based on these broad categories, is also available through the International Society for the Study of Vascular Anomalies (ISSVA Classification of Vascular Anomalies 2014, issva.org/classification).

Although other vascular tumors are rare in children, oral and maxillofacial surgeons may encounter them frequently. The giant cell lesion (GCL), pyogenic granuloma, and aneurysmal bone cyst (ABC) are not considered true vascular neoplasms, but have a strong vascular component, and therefore, they will be discussed here.

HEMANGIOMA
Epidemiology

Hemangiomas are the most common vascular lesions of infancy and are found in the head and neck in 40% to 60% of cases.[2,3] The incidence is between 3% and 10% by the age of 1 year and is more common in premature infants, girls, and Caucasians.[4–6] Skin lesions are the most frequent

[a] Hôpital de l'Enfant-Jésus, Centre Hospitalier Universitaire de Québec, Laval University, Québec, Québec, Canada; [b] Department of Oral and Maxillofacial Surgery, Massachusetts General Hospital, Boston, MA, USA; [c] Department of Oral and Maxillofacial Surgery, Massachusetts General Hospital, Harvard School of Dental Medicine, Boston, MA, USA
* Corresponding author.
E-mail address: carlbchrd@gmail.com

Oral Maxillofacial Surg Clin N Am 28 (2016) 105–113
http://dx.doi.org/10.1016/j.coms.2015.07.010
1042-3699/16/$ – see front matter © 2016 Elsevier Inc. All rights reserved.

area of involvement, but these can be seen in internal organs, such as the liver, brain, and gastrointestinal tract (**Figs. 1** and **2**).[7] They are usually solitary, but multiple lesions are seen in 20% of cases.[2] If more than 4 cutaneous lesions are found, it is suggested to assess for internal lesions. Hemangiomas of the liver can result in life-threatening bleeding.[2] Large lesions of the face combined with other vascular anomalies should prompt suspicion of PHACE syndrome (*P*osterior fossa malformations, *H*emangiomas, *A*rterial lesions, *C*ardiac abnormalities [coarctation of the aorta], and *E*ye anomalies).[2,3,8]

Origin

Hemangiomas are composed of hyperplastic endothelial cells exhibiting increased mitotic activity.[1] The cause remains incompletely understood, although an autosomal transmission is presumed.[7] Two proangiogenic factors are involved during the proliferative phase: fibroblast growth factor (FGF) and vascular endothelial growth factors (VEGF),[9] which is important because it explains, in part, the efficacy of β-adrenergic receptor-blocking agent to treat these lesions (see Treatment section).[10]

Evolution

Cutaneous hemangiomas may not be visible at birth, but can present as a subtle erythematous macula or papule in up to 40% of cases.[1,11] They become more apparent within the first 6 weeks of life and then undergo a proliferative phase

during the subsequent year.[11] Some lesions may have a late proliferative phase, starting later and lasting longer. During this phase, increased endothelial activity and hyperplasia are noted. After proliferation, involution of the tumor occurs over the next several years (up to age 7), a phenomenon not observed with vascular malformations.[11] At this stage, cellular activity is characterized by apoptosis of endothelial cells and decreased angiogenesis.[1] The abnormal vascular channels are replaced with fat and fibrous tissue. Different phases may be present within the same lesion. A lesion completely mature at birth that does not undergo a proliferative phase is called a congenital hemangioma.

Clinical Appearance

The clinical appearance may vary depending on the depth of the tumor. The classic bright red strawberry-like appearance may not be evident if the lesion is situated deeper into the subcutaneous tissues. It can then be misdiagnosed as a vascular malformation, with the overlying skin exhibiting a normal appearance. In the past, superficial lesions were referred to as capillary hemangiomas, and deep lesions were referred to as cavernous hemangiomas.[1] These terms should be reserved for histologic description, because they have no bearing on clinical behavior or treatment. Tumors combining superficial and deeper parts (compound) are also encountered.

In a retrospective chart review of 445 children referred for biopsy of cervical masses, Torsiglieri

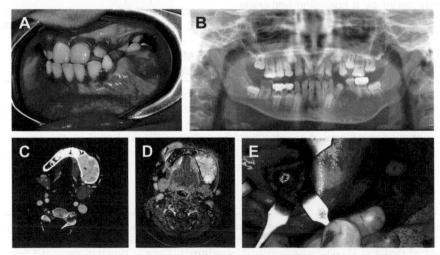

Fig. 1. Intraoral photograph (*A*) of an 11-year-old male patient referred for a vestibular mass of the left mandible. The panoramic radiograph (*B*) shows a poorly defined expansile multilocular lesion with displacement of teeth. Computed tomography angiography (*C*) and MRI (*D*) confirmed the suspected diagnosis of intraosseous hemangioma. The lesion was successfully embolized and enucleated (*E*) without complications or recurrence.

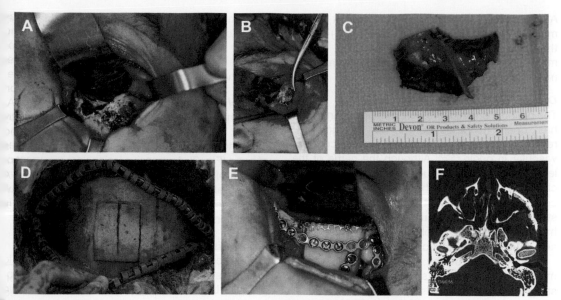

Fig. 2. Intraoperative pictures (*A, B*) of a residual hemangioma of the left zygomatic bone on a 44-year-old female patient referred for facial pain. An en-bloc resection (*C*) was realized and the residual defect was reconstructed with a parietal bone graft (*D, E*). Postoperative axial CT scan view of the reconstruction (*F*).

and colleagues[12] found that only 2% were hemangiomas. This 2% underestimates the incidence, because many hemangiomas can be diagnosed based on appearance alone, without the need for a biopsy.

Diagnosis

The diagnosis is usually established with a thorough history and physical examination, without the need for further imaging.[13] Ultrasound, MRI, or angiography can be helpful in the diagnosis of large, internal, and deep tumors.

Treatment

As most lesions do involute spontaneously, close observation and reassurance is all that is necessary. More aggressive lesions, or those in dangerous areas (airway compromise), may require intervention during the proliferative phase to prevent deformity and potentially prevent negative psychological impact. A variety of treatment modalities have been proposed for hemangiomas, including corticosteroid and interferon-α-2a (IFN-α-2a) or IFN-α-2b injection, surgical removal, and laser treatment.[2,4,14]

Recently, reports of successful treatment with antiadrenergic agents have changed the approach to these lesions. In 2008, Léauté-Labrèze and colleagues[9] first reported the successful treatment of 11 children with problematic hemangiomas with a nonselective β-adrenergic blocker (propanolol). Several other studies have reported similar observations with systemic propranolol.[15–20] Different hypotheses for the efficacy of this treatment have been proposed, including vasoconstriction, decreased levels of VEGF and FGF, and apoptosis of endothelial cells. Recently, a multicenter randomized controlled trial on 456 patients showed successful results in 88% of hemangiomas treated with propanolol compared with 5% with the placebo. The ideal dose has been shown to be 3 mg/kg/day for a period of 6 months.[20]

Surgical treatment of hemangiomas is limited to the removal of residual fibrofatty tissue, nonresponding lesions to pharmaceutical treatment, and tumors of the face at risk of causing severe deformation (ie, those affecting the nose and eyelids) or with a contraindication to the use of adrenergic blockade.[14,21]

Complications

Complications are uncommon with most hemangiomas; however, larger tumors can bleed, or become ulcerated or infected. The use of the pulse-dye laser may be beneficial with superficial lesions and ulcerations. Bleeding can usually be managed with compression dressings.

LESIONS WITH PROMINENT VASCULAR COMPONENT
Giant Cell Lesions

Epidemiology
The giant cell lesion (GCL) is a benign osseous tumor that affects the maxillofacial skeleton.

Although rare in the general population, it occurs more commonly in women and girls (2:1) and in the first and second decade of life.[22–26] The mandible is more frequently affected than the maxilla.[27]

Origin

The biologic origin of the GCL remains unknown. It has been hypothesized to be inflammatory, resembling sarcoidosis, as well as endocrine, or vascular in origin.[28–30] Although the name of the lesion refers to the frequent presence of multinucleated giant cells in the tumor, the neoplastic cell is generally thought to be the mononuclear stromal cell.[31] The multinucleated giant cells have been shown to be phenotypically osteoclasts and activated by the stromal cells.[32]

Although controversy exists, the GCL of the maxillofacial skeleton seems to exist on the same spectrum of disease as the giant cell tumor of the axial/appendicular skeleton.[22–24] Contributing to the confusion is the various terminologies used over the years. The GCL of the maxillofacial skeleton has been referred to as a central giant cell reparative granuloma, given reports of its spontaneous regression, but is generally destructive. It is not a granulomatous lesion resulting

from an inciting agent. Comparing maxillofacial lesions to the classic giant cell tumor axial/appendicular lesions, using clinical and radiographic criteria as well as histology, showed little to no difference.[33,34]

Clinical appearance

GCLs have varying clinical behavior and appearance.[27] Nonaggressive GCLs are small and asymptomatic and do not disturb teeth or cortices of bone (**Fig. 3**). Aggressive lesions are recurrent or meet 3 of the following 5 criteria: are painful, are large in size (>5 cm), exhibit rapid growth, result in thinned/perforated cortices, and result in resorption of teeth.[27]

Diagnosis

The clinical and radiographic appearance should prompt suspicion in the proper patient demographic, but is not diagnostic. The lesion should be classified as aggressive or nonaggressive and biopsy is necessary. A GCL in situ is often a brown color, resembling the brown tumor of hyperparathyroidism. Although it is quite friable, it is easily separated from the surrounding bone. Given its prominent vascular component, bleeding can be significant.

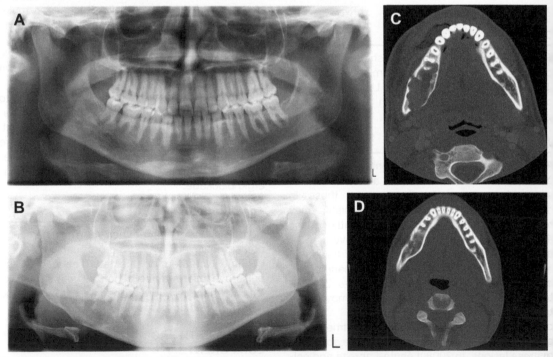

Fig. 3. Preoperative panoramic radiograph (*A*) and CT scan (*B*) of a large right mandibular aggressive GCL with erosion of teeth and lingual cortical plate perforation. The patient was treated successfully with simple enucleation, preserving teeth and inferior alveolar nerve and IFN-α-2a (3 million units/m²) for 9 months. One-year postoperative CT scan (*C*) shows complete bone fill, and 9-year postoperative panoramic radiograph (*D*) shows no recurrence.

Histopathologic findings consist of multinucleated giant cells among a prominent mononuclear stroma. Prominent vessels and hemosiderin are seen. It is not possible to distinguish an aggressive versus nonaggressive lesion histologically.[27,34,35]

Treatment

Although reports of spontaneous regression exist, GCLs are more commonly destructive and require operative management. The gold standard for aggressive lesions remains en-bloc resection, but it is used sparingly given the benign nature of the tumor. Alternative, less-invasive treatment options have been developed. No consensus exists regarding the best treatment at least partly due to the wide range of clinical behavior and overall lack of understanding of the biologic origin. Beyond clinical and radiographic criteria at the time of diagnosis, no biomarker exists to predict behavior particularly for intermediate lesions (ie, those aggressive appearing but not meeting criteria).[36]

Nonaggressive GCLs typically respond to enucleation and curettage alone with low recurrence rate. Adjacent structures such as teeth or the inferior alveolar nerve can be spared. Aggressive lesions have a high recurrence rate with enucleation and curettage alone.

As aggressive lesions can display rapid growth and prominent vascular component, it has been hypothesized that aggressive lesions are the osseous equivalent to the infantile hemangioma.[30] Therefore, IFN-α-2b with its antiangiogenic effects has been used as an adjuvant for aggressive lesions. In this protocol, aggressive GCLs are curetted, leaving surrounding structures such as teeth and the inferior alveolar nerve undisturbed, followed by a subcutaneous injection of IFN-α-2b (3 million units/m^2 of body surface area) until the lesion has filled with bone (typically 10–12 months). No recurrences were found in 26 patients treated with this protocol.[37] The disadvantage of this treatment has been the associated side effects of IFN-α-2a. Fever and flulike symptoms can occur 24 to 48 hours after the initial dose, but only 15% have side effects requiring cessation of therapy.[37]

The close resemblance of the lesions to the brown tumor of hyperparathyroidism has prompted the use of calcitonin as adjuvant and primary treatment of GCLs.[29,38,39] Subcutaneous injection of calcitonin has been effective for both nonaggressive and aggressive lesions.[38] The main disadvantage is the delay in response to treatment, which can be prohibitive in rapidly growing lesions.

The use of intralesional steroids has been reported with varying success rates.[28,40,41] This technique is most effective for small unilocular lesions, but success has also been reported in larger aggressive lesions.[42]

Recently, the receptor activator of nuclear kappa-B ligand (RANK-L;Denosumab) has had some success in both axial-appendicular and maxillofacial GCLs with and without operative intervention[42,43]; this is based on the prominent role of the pathway in osteoclast-mediated bone resorption. Denosumab is not currently recommended for the skeletally immature pediatric patient, which represents a large portion of maxillofacial GCLs. Additional studies are needed to determine the role of Denosumab in the management of maxillofacial GCLs.

Pyogenic Granuloma

Pyogenic granulomas (PG) are not vascular neoplasms, but are composed of a highly vascular proliferation resembling a reactive granuloma.[44] It has also been called lobular capillary hemangioma by some authors, but this term may be confusing because the behavior and clinical course of a PG is different from hemangiomas.[45] This lesion can be seen in pregnant women and is then termed pregnancy tumor or granuloma gravidarum. Despite being called pyogenic, it is not the result of an infection, but generally a result of trauma or irritation.

The vast majority of PG lesions are present in the head and neck. In a review of 178 cases of PG, Patrice and colleagues[45] found that 62.4% of lesions were in the head and neck, 19.7% on the trunk, 12.9% on the upper extremities, and 5.0% on the lower extremities.

Intraoral lesions are seen most commonly on the gingiva (75%), but can also be found on the tongue, lips, and mucosal surfaces.[46] It is common in children and young adults and has a female predilection. They are seen more often on the maxilla and anteriorly in the oral cavity. They have a bright red appearance and sometimes ulcerate or bleed (Fig. 4). Chronic lesions can become hyperkeratotic and less erythematous or prone to bleeding.

PGs are easily treated by complete surgical excision.[47] If caused by chronic irritation, removal of the causative agent is also necessary to avoid recurrence. Complete removal of gingival lesions may result in periodontal defects. The use of Er:-YAG laser may reduce bleeding and postoperative pain, but has not been shown to be superior in preventing recurrence.[47,48]

Aneurysmal Bone Cyst

Aneurysmal bon cyst (ABC) is a benign neoplasm that infrequently affects the craniofacial skeleton.

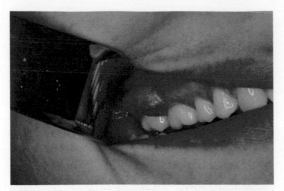

Fig. 4. Intraoral photograph of a right maxillary pyogenic granuloma.

Despite the implication of its name, it is neither a vascular aneurysm nor a bone cyst.[49] It represents 1.5% of nonodontogenic jaw tumors, but is far more frequent in the axial and appendicular skeleton.[50] It affects individuals younger than 30 years, and females predominantly.[51] They are more common in the mandible than the maxilla, with the highest prevalence in the regions of the mandibular body, angle, and ramus.[52]

Although several theories exist, its origin remains unknown. Some think that the lesions are the result of an arteriovenous malformation, causing bleeding and expansion of bone. Others have proposed a traumatic cause, given the predilection for the mandible; however, many patients do not report such a history, and lesions are typically asymptomatic. Between 20% and 30% of patients with an ABC have a concomitant neoplasm, such as a GCL or other fibro-osseous lesion, and are given the term ABC-Plus.[50] This finding has led some to hypothesize that ABCs are the result of a hemorrhagic bony expansion caused by bleeding of a neoplasm, sometimes completely destroying any evidence of the original lesion, and leaving only the aneurysmal anomaly.[50,53]

Radiographically, ABCs appear as unilocular or multilocular radiolucencies with cortical thinning and expansion. Microscopic examination will reveal blood-filled cavities, without endothelial lining, surrounded with fibrous connective tissue and multinucleated giant cells.[51]

If not associated with other lesions, recurrence rates as high as 60% have been reported with enucleation and curettage alone,[50,54] possibly due to incomplete curettage, or to the unrecognized presence of other neoplasms (ABC-Plus). Enucleation, with supplemental cryotherapy, seems to provide improved results, with only an 8% recurrence observed.[54] When other lesions are present, the treatment should be selected to eradicate both lesions, and this may require en-bloc resection.[50]

RARE VASCULAR LESIONS
Kaposiform Hemangioendothelioma and Tufted Angioma

Kaposiform hemangioendothelioma (KHE) is a rare lesion of endothelial cells that is similar to hemangiomas and Kaposi's sarcoma.[55] Very few cases have been reported in the literature. They are not common in the head and neck area and usually appear before the age of 1 year. The clinical presentation is similar to a hemangioma, but without the typical involution phase.

Tufted angioma (TA) is also an anomaly of endothelial cells. Its name comes from the typical tufted organization of the endothelial cells. TAs appear as an erythematous macule or plaque on the skin of the trunk, extremities, and head and neck area. Mucosal involvement has been reported.[56]

The Kasabach-Merritt phenomenon (KMP) is a complication associated with KHE and TA. It is characterized by the presence of a large vascular lesion, thrombocytopenia, and a consumption coagulopathy, causing significant bleeding, and it must be treated aggressively. It was originally thought to be a complication of hemangiomas, but it is now known that KHE and TA are associated with KMP.

Juvenile Nasopharyngeal Angiofibroma

Juvenile nasopharyngeal angiofibroma (JNA) is a benign, highly vascular tumor of the nasospharynx that can be locally aggressive and destructive. It represents 0.05% to 0.5% of all head and neck tumors.[57] The classic presentation is a unilateral nasopharyngeal mass that results in nasal obstruction and epistaxis.[58] JNA often originates in the area of the sphenopalatine foramen, before progressing into the nose and pterygomaxillary space.[58] It is seen almost exclusively in male adolescents. A hormonal influence has been theorized, but remains unclear.[59]

The lesion is composed of numerous thin-walled blood vessels surrounded by connective tissue. Surgical access is difficult and may explain the high recurrence rate (26%–46%) with local excision.[57] Transfacial, intraoral (transpalatal, Le Fort I), and endonasal endoscopic techniques have all been described for the surgical removal of JNA.[60] The technique is selected based on location and amount of tissue invasion. Preoperative embolization is helpful in reducing intraoperative bleeding and can potentially reduce recurrences by improving visualization.[57]

SUMMARY

Oral and maxillofacial surgeons should be involved in the multidisciplinary team approach to treat ascular lesions in the pediatric age group. Vascular lesions are common in the head and neck area and can cause facial disfigurement. The efficacy of propanolol to treat problematic hemangiomas has considerably changed the approach to these lesions.

Similarly to hemangiomas, the biology of GCLs is not completely understood, and the use of pharmaceutical agents has shown promising results. This approach is particularly interesting in children, because aggressive surgical procedures could affect facial growth and cause deformation.

REFERENCES

1. Mulliken JB, Glowacki J. Hemangiomas and vascular malformations in infants and children: a classification based on endothelial characteristics. Plast Reconstr Surg 1982;69:412.
2. Smith SP Jr, Buckingham ED, Williams EF 3rd. Management of cutaneous juvenile hemangiomas. Facial Plast Surg 2008;24:50.
3. Hoff SR, Rastatter JC, Richter GT. Head and neck vascular lesions. Otolaryngol Clin North Am 2015; 48:29.
4. Frieden IJ, Eichenfield LF, Esterly NB, et al. Guidelines of care for hemangiomas of infancy. American Academy of Dermatology Guidelines/Outcomes Committee. J Am Acad Dermatol 1997;37:631.
5. Kilcline C, Frieden IJ. Infantile hemangiomas: how common are they? A systematic review of the medical literature. Pediatr Dermatol 2008;25:168.
6. Munden A, Butschek R, Tom WL, et al. Prospective study of infantile haemangiomas: incidence, clinical characteristics and association with placental anomalies. Br J Dermatol 2014;170:907.
7. Mulliken JB, Fishman SJ, Burrows PE. Vascular anomalies. Curr Probl Surg 2000;37:517.
8. Bellaud G, Puzenat E, Billon-Grand NC, et al. PHACE syndrome, a series of six patients: clinical and morphological manifestations, propranolol efficacy, and safety. Int J Dermatol 2015;54:102.
9. Léauté-Labrèze C, Dumas de la Roque E, Hubiche T, et al. Propranolol for severe hemangiomas of infancy. N Engl J Med 2008;358:2649.
10. Leaute-Labreze C, Hoeger P, Mazereeuw-Hautier J, et al. A randomized, controlled trial of oral propranolol in infantile hemangioma. N Engl J Med 2015; 372:735.
11. Chang LC, Haggstrom AN, Drolet BA, et al. Growth characteristics of infantile hemangiomas: implications for management. Pediatrics 2008;122:360.
12. Torsiglieri AJ Jr, Tom LW, Ross AJ 3rd, et al. Pediatric neck masses: guidelines for evaluation. Int J Pediatr Otorhinolaryngol 1988;16:199.
13. Griauzde J, Srinivasan A. Imaging of vascular lesions of the head and neck. Radiol Clin North Am 2015;53:197.
14. Bauland CG, Luning TH, Smit JM, et al. Untreated hemangiomas: growth pattern and residual lesions. Plast Reconstr Surg 2011;127:1643.
15. Sans V, de la Roque ED, Berge J, et al. Propranolol for severe infantile hemangiomas: follow-up report. Pediatrics 2009;124:e423.
16. Izadpanah A, Izadpanah A, Kanevsky J, et al. Propranolol versus corticosteroids in the treatment of infantile hemangioma: a systematic review and meta-analysis. Plast Reconstr Surg 2013;131:601.
17. Bertrand J, McCuaig C, Dubois J, et al. Propranolol versus prednisone in the treatment of infantile hemangiomas: a retrospective comparative study. Pediatr Dermatol 2011;28:649.
18. Price CJ, Lattouf C, Baum B, et al. Propranolol vs corticosteroids for infantile hemangiomas: a multicenter retrospective analysis. Arch Dermatol 2011; 147:1371.
19. Hogeling M, Adams S, Wargon O. A randomized controlled trial of propranolol for infantile hemangiomas. Pediatrics 2011;128:e259.
20. Leaute-Labreze C, Dumas de la Roque E, Nacka F, et al. Double-blind randomized pilot trial evaluating the efficacy of oral propranolol on infantile haemangiomas in infants < 4 months of age. Br J Dermatol 2013;169:181.
21. Eivazi B, Werner JA. Management of vascular malformations and hemangiomas of the head and neck–an update. Curr Opin Otolaryngol Head Neck Surg 2013;21:157.
22. Austin LT Jr, Dahlin DC, Royer RQ. Giant-cell reparative granuloma and related conditions affecting the jawbones. Oral Surg Oral Med Oral Pathol 1959;12:1285.
23. Auclair PL, Cuenin P, Kratochvil FJ, et al. A clinical and histomorphologic comparison of the central giant cell granuloma and the giant cell tumor. Oral Surg Oral Med Oral Pathol 1988;66:197.
24. Waldron CA, Shafer WG. The central giant cell reparative granuloma of the jaws. An analysis of 38 cases. Am J Clin Pathol 1966;45:437.
25. Eisenbud L, Stern M, Rothberg M, et al. Central giant cell granuloma of the jaws: experiences in the management of thirty-seven cases. J Oral Maxillofac Surg 1988;46:376.
26. Sidhu MS, Parkash H, Sidhu SS. Central giant cell granuloma of jaws–review of 19 cases. Br J Oral Maxillofac Surg 1995;33:43.
27. Chuong R, Kaban LB, Kozakewich H, et al. Central giant cell lesions of the jaws: a clinicopathologic study. J Oral Maxillofac Surg 1986;44:708.
28. Terry B, Jacoway J. Management of central giant cell lesions: an alternative to surgical therapy. Oral Maxillofacial Surg Clin N Am 1994;44:579–600.

29. Harris M. Central giant cell granulomas of the jaws regress with calcitonin therapy. Br J Oral Maxillofac Surg 1993;31:89.

30. Kaban LB, Mulliken JB, Ezekowitz RA, et al. Antiangiogenic therapy of a recurrent giant cell tumor of the mandible with interferon alfa-2a. Pediatrics 1999;103:1145.

31. Itonaga I, Hussein I, Kudo O, et al. Cellular mechanisms of osteoclast formation and lacunar resorption in giant cell granuloma of the jaw. J Oral Pathol Med 2003;32:224.

32. Flanagan AM, Nui B, Tinkler SM, et al. The multinucleate cells in giant cell granulomas of the jaw are osteoclasts. Cancer 1988;62:1139.

33. Resnick CM, Margolis J, Susarla SM, et al. Maxillofacial and axial/appendicular giant cell lesions: unique tumors or variants of the same disease?– A comparison of phenotypic, clinical, and radiographic characteristics. J Oral Maxillofac Surg 2010;68:130.

34. Peacock ZS, Resnick CM, Susarla SM, et al. Do histologic criteria predict biologic behavior of giant cell lesions? J Oral Maxillofac Surg 2012;70:2573.

35. Ficarra G, Kaban LB, Hansen LS. Central giant cell lesions of the mandible and maxilla: a clinicopathologic and cytometric study. Oral Surg Oral Med Oral Pathol 1987;64:44.

36. Dewsnup NC, Susarla SM, Abulikemu M, et al. Immunohistochemical evaluation of giant cell tumors of the jaws using CD34 density analysis. J Oral Maxillofac Surg 2008;66:928.

37. Kaban LB, Troulis MJ, Wilkinson MS, et al. Adjuvant antiangiogenic therapy for giant cell tumors of the jaws. J Oral Maxillofac Surg 2007;65:2018.

38. Pogrel MA. Calcitonin therapy for central giant cell granuloma. J Oral Maxillofac Surg 2003;61:649.

39. de Lange J, van den Akker HP, Veldhuijzen van Zanten GO, et al. Calcitonin therapy in central giant cell granuloma of the jaw: a randomized double-blind placebo-controlled study. Int J Oral Maxillofac Surg 2006;35:791.

40. Carlos R, Sedano HO. Intralesional corticosteroids as an alternative treatment for central giant cell granuloma. Oral Surg Oral Med Oral Pathol Oral Radiol Endod 2002;93:161.

41. Nogueira RL, Teixeira RC, Cavalcante RB, et al. Intralesional injection of triamcinolone hexacetonide as an alternative treatment for central giant-cell granuloma in 21 cases. Int J Oral Maxillofac Surg 2010;39:1204.

42. Chawla S, Henshaw R, Seeger L, et al. Safety and efficacy of denosumab for adults and skeletally mature adolescents with giant cell tumour of bone: interim analysis of an open-label, parallel-group, phase 2 study. Lancet Oncol 2013;14:901.

43. Schreuder WH, Coumou AW, Kessler PA, et al. Alternative pharmacologic therapy for aggressive central

giant cell granuloma: denosumab. J Oral Maxillofac Surg 2014;72:1301.

44. Neville BW, Damm DD, Allen CM, et al. Soft tissue tumors. In: Neville BW, Damm DD, Allen CM, et al, editors. Oral and maxillofacial pathology. 2nd edition. St Louis (MO): Elsevier; 2009. p. 447.

45. Patrice SJ, Wiss K, Mulliken JB. Pyogenic granuloma (lobular capillary hemangioma): a clinicopathologic study of 178 cases. Pediatr Dermatol 1991; 8:267.

46. Zain RB, Khoo SP, Yeo JF. Oral pyogenic granuloma (excluding pregnancy tumour)–a clinical analysis of 304 cases. Singapore Dent J 1995;20:8.

47. Bhaskar SN, Jacoway JR. Pyogenic granuloma–clinical features, incidence, histology, and result of treatment: report of 242 cases. J Oral Surg 1966; 24:391.

48. Fekrazad R, Nokhbatolfoghahaei H, Khoei F, et al. Pyogenic granuloma: surgical treatment with Er:YAG laser. J Lasers Med Sci 2014;5:199.

49. Bataineh AB. Aneurysmal bone cysts of the maxilla: a clinicopathologic review. J Oral Maxillofac Surg 1997;55:1212.

50. Padwa BL, Denhart BC, Kaban LB. Aneurysmal bone cyst-"plus": a report of three cases. J Oral Maxillofac Surg 1997;55:1144.

51. Neville BW, Damm DD, Allen CM, et al. Bone pathology. In: Neville BW, Damm DD, Allen CM, et al, editors. Oral and maxillofacial pathology. St Louis (MO): Elsevier; 2009. p. 533.

52. Trent C, Byl FM. Aneurysmal bone cyst of the mandible. Ann Otol Rhinol Laryngol 1993;102:917.

53. Bernier JL, Bhaskar SN. Aneurysmal bone cysts of the mandible. Oral Surg Oral Med Oral Pathol 1958;11:1018.

54. Kershisnik M, Batsakis JG. Aneurysmal bone cysts of the jaws. Ann Otol Rhinol Laryngol 1994;103:164.

55. Mukerji SS, Osborn AJ, Roberts J, et al. Kaposiform hemangioendothelioma (with Kasabach Merritt syndrome) of the head and neck: case report and review of the literature. Int J Pediatr Otorhinolaryngol 2009;73:1474.

56. da Silva AD, Ramos Gde O, Gomes RF, et al. Tufted angioma in children: report of two cases and a review of the literature. Case Rep Dent 2014;2014: 942489.

57. Lutz J, Holtmannspotter M, Flatz W, et al. Preoperative embolization to improve the surgical management and outcome of juvenile nasopharyngeal angiofibroma (JNA) in a single center: 10-year experience. Clin Neuroradiol 2015. [Epub ahead of print].

58. Khoueir N, Nicolas N, Rohayem Z, et al. Exclusive endoscopic resection of juvenile nasopharyngeal angiofibroma: a systematic review of the literature. Otolaryngol Head Neck Surg 2014; 150:350.

59. Liu Z, Wang J, Wang H, et al. Hormonal receptors and vascular endothelial growth factor in juvenile nasopharyngeal angiofibroma: immunohistochemical and tissue microarray analysis. Acta Otolaryngol 2015;135:51.

60. Kopec T, Borucki L, Szyfter W. Fully endoscopic resection of juvenile nasopharyngeal angiofibroma—own experience and clinical outcomes. Int J Pediatr Otorhinolaryngol 2014;78:1015.

Strategies to Overcome Late Complications from Radiotherapy for Childhood Head and Neck Cancers

Michael T. Spiotto, MD, PhD[a,b,*], Philip P. Connell, MD[c]

KEYWORDS

- Radiotherapy • Intensity-modulated radiotherapy • Proton therapy • Radiation-induced neoplasms
- Image-guided radiotherapy

KEY POINTS

- Radiotherapy is administered with increasing frequency given the increasing rates of pediatric head and neck cancer and improved long-term survival rates.
- Long-term radiation morbidities include abnormal tooth development and decay, bone and soft tissue hypoplasia, hypopituitarism, and damage to visual and auditory organs.
- Radiation increases the risk of second malignancies, which are associated with adverse outcomes.
- Approaches have been developed to reduce the risk of late radiation toxicities, including improvements in the delivery of radiation that more precisely targets tumors and that uses newer technologies, including proton beam therapy and image-guided radiotherapy.

INTRODUCTION: THE PROBLEM OF RADIATION MORBIDITIES IN CHILDREN

Even though pediatric cancer is the second leading cause of death in children aged 5 to 14 years,[1] the 5-year overall survival for childhood cancers has increased to 83% for patients diagnosed from 2003 to 2009 compared with 56% for those diagnosed from 1974 to 1976.[2,3] Of the children surviving 5 years or more, approximately 80% were treated with radiotherapy.[4] Furthermore, radiotherapy for head and neck pediatric cancers is becoming increasingly common, as shown by an analysis of the National Cancer Institute's Surveillance, Epidemiology, and End Results (SEER).

This analysis showed that the incidence of pediatric head and neck cancers (overall 12% of all pediatric cancers) was increasing faster than pediatric cancers overall.[5] For cancers involving the head and neck area, the most common pathologic types include lymphomas (Hodgkin lymphoma and non-Hodgkin lymphoma); neural tumors (neuroblastoma and retinoblastoma); and soft tissue sarcomas, including rhabdomyosarcomas.[5]

Because various types of pediatric cancers can arise in the head and neck region, radiation treatments vary widely based on the histologic type and site of disease. Specific cancer types are treated with different radiation doses, and the

Disclosure: The authors have nothing to disclose.
[a] Department of Radiation and Cellular Oncology, University of Chicago Medical Center, KCBD 6142, 900 East 57th Street, Chicago, IL 60637, USA; [b] Department of Radiation Oncology, University of Illinois at Chicago Medical Center, 1801 W. Taylor Street, Chicago, IL 60612, USA; [c] Department of Radiation and Cellular Oncology, University of Chicago Medical Center, 5758 South Maryland Avenue, MC 9006, Suite 1D, Chicago, IL 60637, USA
* Corresponding author. Department of Radiation and Cellular Oncology, The University of Chicago, KCBD 6142, 900 East 57th Street, Chicago, IL 60637.
E-mail address: mspiotto@radonc.uchicago.edu

Oral Maxillofacial Surg Clin N Am 28 (2016) 115–126
http://dx.doi.org/10.1016/j.coms.2015.07.009
1042-3699/16/$ – see front matter © 2016 Elsevier Inc. All rights reserved.

intensity of the dose is a major determinant of long-term treatment-related morbidities. Radiation doses are prescribed in units of Gray (Gy), which denotes the amount of energy that is absorbed per unit mass in the radiated tissue. Radiation doses tend to be low (usually <15 Gy) for patients with leukemia receiving total body irradiation (TBI) in preparation for stem cell transplantation. Likewise, doses tend to be low (generally 20–40 Gy) in lymphomas and neuroblastomas, which require localized radiotherapy to specific disease sites. Nonetheless, these patients are at risk for developing hypopituitarism, cataracts, and secondary cancers. By contrast, soft tissue sarcomas and other solid tumors, such as squamous cell carcinomas, require considerably higher radiation doses of 50 Gy or more. In these cases, patients are at risk for dental damage, bone hypoplasia, and hearing and vision toxicities.

Given these risks, this article reviews approaches to minimize the toxicities from pediatric head and neck radiotherapy. The first part of this article discusses current and emerging approaches to minimize radiation-induced toxicities. The second part discusses the long-term morbidities from radiation therapy, specifically addressing the recent advances that minimize these risks of head and neck radiotherapy in children.

THERAPEUTIC OPTIONS TO MINIMIZE RADIATION MORBIDITIES

Several groups have sought to reduce the risks of late radiation morbidities by using modalities such as proton beam radiotherapy (PBR) and intensity-modulated radiotherapy (IMRT). Compared with conventional radiotherapy, these modalities offer the potential to deliver radiation plans that better conform to the targeted tumor. Image-guidance techniques ensure more reproducible delivery of radiation plans. In addition, medical approaches such as radiation protectors

and mitigators may help to minimize radiation toxicities. These approaches to avoid radiation toxicities in pediatric patients with cancer are detailed later.

Overview of Radiation Therapy and Planning

The radiation therapy planning process begins by defining the tumor target and susceptible normal tissues. The process then involves arranging the radiation beams such that they cover target tissues while minimizing exposure to the adjacent normal organs. Radiation therapy planning begins with a process called simulation, which uses computed tomography (CT) to image the patient and tumor. Secondary imaging studies including MRI and PET scans are aligned with the treatment-planning CT in order to delineate the tumor target, which is termed gross tumor volume (GTV; see red outline, Fig. 1). Additional margins are included to account for microscopic tumor spread, resulting in an expanded structure termed the clinical target volume (CTV). An additional volumetric expansion is added to account for daily variations in tumor motion and in patient positioning, which is termed the planning target volume (PTV; magenta outline Fig. 2). The physician then works with dosimetrists and medical physicists to develop an optimal radiation delivery plan, optimally covering the tumor target and minimizing dose to the normal organs (see Fig. 2). The resulting plan is used to deliver a prescribed radiation dose.

Radiation Modalities: Protons Versus Photons

Pediatric cancers have been treated with photon-based radiotherapy using three-dimensional (3D) conformal radiotherapy (3D-CRT) or IMRT and more recently, with proton-based therapy. Photon radiotherapy likely provides more skin sparing compared with traditional proton beams. By contrast, proton therapy probably provides more

Contrast enhanced T1 MRI

Treatment planning CT

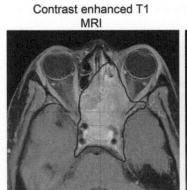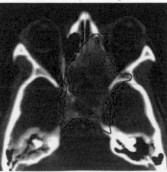

Fig. 1. Radiation therapy planning to define radiation therapy targets. A pediatric patient with a parameningeal rhabdomyosarcoma and brain invasion underwent radiation therapy simulation consisting of treatment-planning CT. The contrast enhanced MRI was fused to the treatment-planning CT. The GTV is delineated in the red outline using both the MRI and treatment planning CT images.

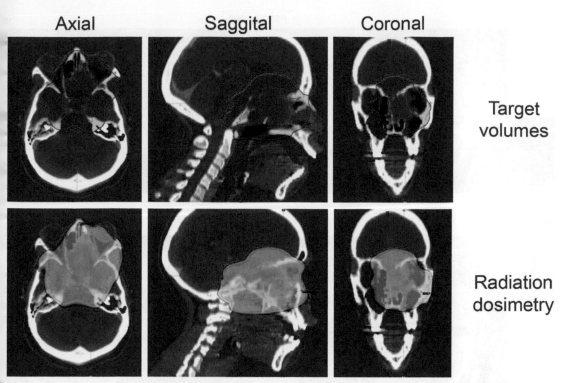

Axial	Saggital	Coronal	
			Target volumes
			Radiation dosimetry

Fig. 2. IMRT planning for rhabdomyosarcoma. Upper row depicts the orthogonal views of the planning volumes for the patient with parameningeal rhabdomyosarcoma in **Fig. 1.** Red outline depicts the gross tumor. Purple outline depicts the PTV. Lower row depicts the orthogonal views of the radiation dose color wash for an IMRT plan. The dose color wash is set to a minimum dose of 45 Gy.

conformal dose distributions than photon radiotherapy, because of the advantageous physical characteristics of protons. Representative examples of proton and photon radiation dosimetry are shown in **Fig. 3.**

Photon beam radiotherapy has historically depended on 3D-CRT methods for diametric planning; however, more recently IMRT has become commonly used. Compared with 3D-CRT, IMRT enables the radiation beam to better conform to the tumor target by geometrically varying the intensity of the radiation beam in order to better tailored dose distributions to targets while avoiding adjacent normal tissues. IMRT is well suited for cancers such as rhabdomyosarcomas, which require higher radiation doses and reside in close proximity to critical normal structures.[6] Hein and colleagues[7] compared 3D-CRT with IMRT in treating 5 cases of orbital rhabdomyosarcoma. Overall, IMRT reduced radiation exposure to the lens by 26%. However, such protection of critical structures comes at a cost, because more normal tissues receive lower doses of scattered radiation. Compared with 3D-CRT for rhabdomyosarcomas, IMRT generated comparable locoregional control rates of 90% or more at 3 years[8,9] and fewer grade

3 or greater acute toxicities. Therefore, compared with 3D-CRT, IMRT provides similar rates of disease control with less toxicity for pediatric head and neck radiotherapy.

Compared with photon-based radiotherapy, PBR often outperforms 3D-CRT and IMRT in dosimetric sparing of critical structures (see **Fig. 3**). Compared with 3D-CRT for optic gliomas, PBR reduced doses to the contralateral optic nerve, chiasm, pituitary gland, and temporal lobes by 47%, 11%, 13%, and 29%, respectively.[10] Similarly, PBR outperformed 3D-CRT for treating orbital rhabdomyosarcomas.[11] Studying 54 patients with rhabdomyosarcomas, of which half involved the head and neck, Ladra and colleagues[12] showed that PBR significantly improved the normal tissue sparing for 20 of 22 normal structures compared with IMRT. This advantage of PBR compared with IMRT was primarily restricted to tumors located in lateralized sites, whereas tumors located more centrally in the head and neck region had less benefit from PBR. Compared with IMRT, PBR also delivered a 1.8-fold lower integral dose, which is a measure of total radiation dose absorbed by the whole body. In addition, a recent phase II trial showed that PBR provides similar

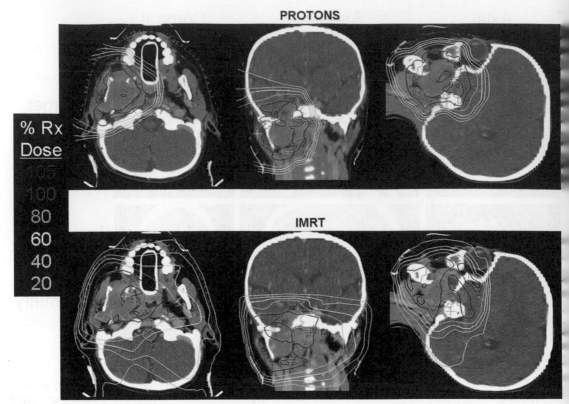

Fig. 3. Comparison of IMRT and proton radiation dosimetry. Representative dosimetry for a 3-field proton treatment plan and a 5-field IMRT plan, with axial, coronal, and sagittal views. The right infratemporal fossa CTV (*thin purple*) and 105% (*maroon*), 100% (*thick red*), 80% (*orange*), 60% (*yellow*), 40% (*light green*) and 20% (*light blue*) isodose lines are shown. In the top panel, the GTV is also depicted (*thin red*). % Rx Dose percent prescribed dose. (*From* Kozak KR, Adams J, Krejcarek SJ, et al. A dosimetric comparison of proton and intensity-modulated photon radiotherapy for pediatric parameningeal rhabdomyosarcomas. Int J Radiat Oncol Biol Phys 2009;74(1):181; with permission.)

disease control and overall survival rates to photon-based radiotherapy.[13] **Table 1** shows the differences in radiation exposure to normal structures in the head and neck region, as a function of radiotherapy type in this study.

Nevertheless, it remains unclear to what extent these PBR-mediated dose reductions (often in the medium and low dose ranges) will translate into clinically significant differences in patient outcomes.[14] Few, if any, studies compared late toxicity rates for proton-based and photon-based radiotherapy. For rhabdomyosarcomas treated with PBR, Ladra and colleagues[13] reported acute grade 3 mucositis in 6% of patients, which is less than the 46% grade 3 or greater mucositis previously reported with 3D-CRT.[15] However, Combs and colleagues[16] reported no grade 3 or greater toxicity in 16 patients treated with IMRT for head and neck rhabdomyosarcoma. Of particular interest are outcomes regarding secondary cancers, especially given

the reduced integral dose with proton beam therapy. Models assessing the risk of secondary cancers have predicted that PBR will reduce the risk of secondary cancers by greater than or equal to 2-fold for rhabdomyosarcomas and 8-fold for medulloblastoma, relative to rates induced with photon-based radiotherapy.[17,18] Although there is no direct comparison of IMRT and PBR for secondary malignancies arising in pediatric cancer survivors, a SEER analysis showed no significant differences in secondary cancers for adult patients.[19] Furthermore, the greater dose conformality of PBR may accentuate some radiation toxicities, such as bone and soft tissue hypoplasia, because of the greater asymmetry in dose distributions.[20] Given the lack of current data, the American Society of Therapeutic Radiation Oncology Emerging technology Committee has not recommend PBR outside of clinical trials for pediatric non–central nervous systems tumors or head and neck cancers.[21] Thus, further studies

Table 1
Comparison of radiation doses to indicated normal tissues using 3D-CRT, IMRT, or PBR for orbital and nonorbital rhabdomyosarcomas

	Radiation Dose (Gy)							
	Orbital				Nonorbital			
	3D-CRT	IMRT	Protons	Ref	3D-CRT	IMRT	Protons	Ref
Brainstem	—	NS	NS	—	36.78	27.08	—	5
					—	26.40	6.9	19
Optic chiasm	—	NS	NS	—	35.25	35.30	—	5
					—	33.30	17.70	19
Pituitary	—	15	4	11	35.89	57.07	28.90	5
						43.40		19
Optic nerve (ipsilateral)	40.0	37	29.2	10	NS	37.3	30.2	19
			31	11				
Optic nerve (contralateral)	7.1	—	0.3	10	NS	30.6	13.9	19
Eye (ipsilateral)	34.2	—	24.7	10	NS	16.4	8.5	19
	—	40	33	11				
Eye (contralateral)	2.9	—	0.3	10	NS	13.3	3.1	19
	—	8	0.1	11				
Lens (ipsilateral)	28.5	—	9.9	10	NS	6.8	1.7	19
	—	32	26	11				
Lens (contralateral)	1.5	—	0.4	10	NS	5.8	0.9	19
	—	3	0	11				
Maxilla	38.5	—	25.0	10	NS	NS	NS	19
	—	12	7	11				

Abbreviation: NS, not stated.
Data from Refs.[5,10,11,19]

are required to address the clinical benefits for PBR.

Efforts to Decrease Radiation Target Volumes with Image Guidance

Radiation toxicities may also be minimized by decreasing the volume of tissue in the radiation field. In order to deliver consistent radiation doses to tumors, the PTV incorporates a setup margin of 0.5 to 1 cm to account for the daily uncertainties in patient positioning. Image-guided radiotherapy (IGRT) is a method that uses frequent imaging before daily radiotherapy fractions in order to improve target localization. IGRT commonly consists of orthogonal diagnostic-quality radiographs and/or cone-beam CT (CBCT) scans. By reducing the uncertainties in patient positioning, this enables reductions in the size of target volumes. From a survey of 7 international institutions with pediatric experience, nearly all cases of head and neck radiotherapy incorporated some form of IGRT for both photon therapy and PBR.[22] Using IGRT, some reports suggest that the setup margin may be reduced to 3.5 mm for patients treated

with weekly CBCT and 2 mm for patients treated with daily CBCT.[23] However, given the paucity of outcome studies using IGRT, reduced setup margins for pediatric head and neck tumors should be applied with caution.

Prevention and Medical Treatment of Radiation-induced Morbidities

The use of systemic radioprotectors such as amifostine may help to limit radiation toxicities. Amifostine is a thiophosphate prodrug that is converted in vivo to a thiol metabolite WR-1065 that scavenges the oxygen free radicals produced by radiation. The radioprotective effect of amifostine is hypothesized to produce a therapeutic advantage by better penetration in normal tissues compared with tumors, which occurs as a result of increased vascular permeability. It may also provide preferential effects in tumors because of an increased alkaline phosphate activity and higher pH in tumors relative to normal tissues. Consensus recommendations suggest that amifostine be considered to reduce radiation-induced xerostomia.[24] Anacak and colleagues[25] showed that subcutaneous amifostine was well tolerated in a small series of 5 children with head and neck cancer treated radiotherapy. Of note, no grade 3 or 4 mucositis or dermatitis occurred even though 4 patients were treated to a high radiation dose (70.2 Gy for nasopharyngeal cancer).

Fewer modalities exist to mitigate late radiation toxicities once they appear. Hyperbaric oxygen (HBO) remains one of the few treatments for radiation-induced osteoradionecrosis and soft tissue damage. HBO likely functions by stimulating angiogenesis and fibroplasia as measured by improved transcutaneous oxygen measurements, histologic assessments, and decreased tissue lactate levels.[26] Ashamalla and colleagues[27] reported on the use of HBO in 10 pediatric patients, of whom 4 were treated with therapeutic HBO for osteoradionecrosis and/or vasculitis. Osteoradionecrosis resolved in all 4 patients and 2 patients showed bone regrowth. Thus, amifostine and HBO may help to avoid or to mitigate radiation morbidities; however, more studies are needed to confirm these activities.

CLINICAL OUTCOMES AND COMPLICATIONS: RADIATION MORBIDITIES

Even though radiotherapy causes both acute and late toxicities, the latter remain the major hurdle in treating pediatric patients with cancer. Acute reactions occur during or shortly after radiotherapy, whereas late effects occur months to years after radiotherapy.[28] Acute effects are most often limited to skin, gastrointestinal tract, and bone marrow; they generally resolve shortly after treatment is completed, given the rapid turnover of specialized cells. By contrast, late effects occur in tissues such as the central nervous system, kidney, and liver; they are generally only partially reversible at best. Late effects represent a culmination of complex processes including stem cell loss, vascular damage, fibrosis, and the loss of slowly dividing parenchymal cells. Although acute radiation-induced toxicities typically resolve within the first few weeks of finishing treatment, late effects appear months to years after treatment. Moreover, the incidence and severity of late effects tend to increase over time. These radiotherapy-related late effects can result in significant personal and societal issues, given that they increase both patient hardship and increased use of health care resources.[29] This article details the toxicities associated with radiation in the pediatric population, including issues with teeth, bone development, hormonal function, hearing, vision, and radiation-induced neoplasms. **Table 2** summarizes the radiation toxicities based on

photon-based or proton-based radiotherapy for rhabdomyosarcomas.[9,11,30–33]

Tooth Development and Decay

Radiation may directly affect dental development depending the patient's age, radiation dose, and specific tooth type. In children with leukemia, Cubukcu and colleagues[34] showed that chemotherapy was associated with abnormal root development in 86.4% of patients, microdontia in 13.5% of patients, and tooth agenesis in 16.2% of patients. Furthermore, the severity of dental disturbances was especially prominent after radiotherapy to the head and neck. Similarly, Sonis and colleagues[35] showed that younger age predicts for increased dental injury after radiotherapy. Even low radiation doses may affect dental development, given that patients treated with TBI before stem cell transplantation showed increased risk of microdontia (56% vs 15%).[36,37] Similarly, Holtta and colleagues[36] showed that patients with neuroblastoma treated with TBI and chemotherapy had a higher dental defect index than patients treated with chemotherapy alone.

In addition to tooth development, radiation predisposes to dental decay by negatively affecting salivary gland function. Radiotherapy causes decreased salivation as well as alterations to the saliva quality, resulting in a thickened, more mucous secretion. Decreased salivation can result in xerostomia (dry mouth), which facilitates bacterial overgrowth in the mouth, changes in pH, and ultimately dental decay. Meazza and colleagues[38] showed that 38% of patients irradiated for head and neck rhabdomyosarcoma developed xerostomia. Using the "Registry for the Evaluation of Side Effects after Radiotherapy in Childhood and Adolescence" (RiSK), Bolling and colleagues[39] showed that acute and late salivary toxicities occurred in salivary glands receiving doses of 20 Gy or more. Concurrent chemotherapy further increases the risk for both acute and late xerostomia. Of note, the radiation tolerance of the salivary glands in pediatric patients is likely similar to that of adults, in that the risk of severe xerostomia is minimized if 1 parotid gland is spared to a mean dose of less than 20 Gy.[40]

In addition, the mastication apparatus, including the jaw, temporomandibular joint (TMJ), and pterygoid and masseter muscles, may be negatively affected by high radiation doses. Children treated to radiation doses of 40 Gy or higher to the TMJ and/or muscles of mastication are at increased risk of trismus or TMJ dysfunction.[41] Furthermore, Mercado and colleagues[42] reported seeing mandibular condyle erosion or sclerosis with doses as low as 30 to 40 Gy. Thus, although lower radiation doses may injure dental development or cause tooth decay, higher radiation doses are associated with dysfunction of the muscles and structures mediating mastication.

Bone and Soft Tissue Hypoplasia

Radiation can also have impacts on bone and soft tissue development, which can be especially problematic for young children receiving higher radiation doses to tumors near the facial bones, or viscerocranium. Extrapolating from radiation effects of long bones, radiation causes bone damage by injuring the blood vessels within the bones, which leads to occlusion of haversian canals and loss of osteocytes. However, the impact of radiation on the viscerocranium remains unclear (compared with long bones), because they have different mechanisms of ossification, embryonic origins, and three-dimensional structures.[43] Guyuron and colleagues[30] defined the threshold radiation dose for adverse effects on bone and soft tissues as 30 Gy and 4 Gy, respectively. Furthermore, young patients (aged <6 years) are more susceptible to these risks, given the degree of bone growth still to come at later ages.

Consequently, bone and soft tissue hypoplasia can cause significant cosmetic morbidities that affect the patient's quality of life with few, if any, corrective options available. Children with craniofacial abnormalities are more likely to have negative social interactions, resulting in worse psychosocial adjustments and lower self-esteem.[44–46] Attempts to correct radiation-induced craniofacial abnormalities with surgical reconstruction are fraught with difficulty because 40% of patients require a second procedure.[47,48] This difficulty in achieving surgical reconstruction stems from the atrophy and fibrosis of the irradiated field, which often precludes the use of local flaps, impairs healing, and increases postoperative complications.[49] Furthermore, these reconstructive surgeries offer only slight improvements in the negative psychosocial consequences occurring in these patients.[45]

Hypopituitarism

Hypopituitarism is a significant sequela that is most commonly associated with disturbances in growth hormone (GH) secretion. Less likely problems include corticotropin, gonadotropin, and thyrotropin hormone deficiencies. Bhandare and colleagues[50] showed that, in 30 patients treated between 20 to 65 Gy, 58% of the patients developed clinical hypopituitarism within 5 years. The

risk factors for developing hypopituitarism include younger ages and higher radiation doses. GH deficiency is typically the initial sign of hypopituitarism; it can be seen after doses as low as 18 Gy, whereas almost all patients receiving 35 Gy or greater displayed abnormalities in GH production. GH deficiency has been associated with decreased height and bone mineralization. By contrast, deficiencies in other pituitary hormones are limited to patients receiving higher radiation doses. For gonadotropins, low pituitary doses ranging from 12 to 24 Gy were associated with precocious puberty, whereas higher radiation doses of more than 40 Gy were associated with gonadotropin deficiencies. These more severe gonadotropin deficiencies prevent children from entering puberty and cause sexual dysfunction in adulthood. Although the median time to develop clinical hypopituitarism is approximately 3 years after radiotherapy,[50] laboratory abnormalities can be observed within months following high-dose radiotherapy to the pituitary. In addition, hypopituitarism is likely related to age of exposure, given that children treated with TBI are more likely to develop hypopituitarism than adults or older children treated with similar TBI regimens.[51,52] Furthermore, Bhandare and colleagues[50] showed that, at 5 years, 90% of patients younger than 10 years of age developed hypopituitarism compared with 38% of children who were older than 10 years of age.

Optic and Hearing Toxicities

Children with orbital tumors are often at risk for complications that impair vision. This finding is especially the case with retinoblastoma and other tumors involving the orbit, wherein visual toxicities include cataracts, conjunctiva keratinization, xerophthalmia, retinopathy, and optic neuropathy. These ocular toxicities have been extensively reviewed by Jeganathan and colleagues.[53] One of the most common toxicities is radiation-induced cataract formation, which can occur after doses as low as 2 Gy. However, cataract extraction corrects vision loss in 68.4% of pediatric patients previously treated for retinoblastoma,[54] although 30.8% of these patients also experience deterioration of vision caused by other radiation side effects, including keratopathy and optic neuropathy. In addition to visual loss, up to 14% of patients developed hearing loss after brain irradiation.[55] Hearing loss strongly depends on the types of chemotherapies used, in addition to the radiation dose received by the cochlea. For mean cochlear doses greater than 45 Gy, there is a greater than 10% chance of high-frequency hearing loss, which

Table 2
Toxicities associated with head and neck radiotherapy for pediatric cancers

Organ Study (Ref)	Photon Radiotherapy	Proton Radiotherapy	Types of Toxicities	Reported Dose When Toxicity Observed
Dental Abnormalities				
IRS II–III[32]	61 out of NR	—	Tooth, agenesis, microdontia, enamel dysplasia, xerostomia, TMJ dysfunction, osteoradionecrosis	20 Gy (odds ratio, 5.6; Ref.[30])
U of Iowa[31]	7 out of 7	—		
MSKCC[8]	—	—		
MGH[10]	—	3 out of 10 (children)		
Craniofacial Malformations				
IRS II–III[32]	74 out of 76	—	Bone and soft tissue hypoplasia	Bone: 30 Gy Soft tissue: 4 Gy (Ref.[29])
U of Iowa[31]	11 out of 15	—		
MSKCC[8]	1 out of 21	—		
MGH[10]	—	7 out of 10		
Hypopituitarism				
GH deficiency				
IRS II–III[32]	36 out of 190	—	Decreased height, decreased bone mineralization	GH: 18 Gy
U of Iowa[31]	6 out of 15	—		
MSKCC[8]	1 out of 21	—		
MGH[10]	—	2 out of 10		
Other Endocrinopathy				
IRS II–III[32]	17 out of 213	—	Delayed puberty, sexual dysfunction, subclinical hypothyroidism	GnRH: 40 Gy ACTH: 24 Gy TSH: 24 Gy
U of Iowa[31]	1 out of 15	—		
MSKCC[8]	—	—		
MGH[10]	—	1 out of 10		

Optic Toxicities			
IRS II-III[32]	45 out of 213	Cataract	2 Gy
U of Iowa[31]	9 out of 11	Keratinization	30 Gy
MSKCC[8]	2 out of 21	Retinopathy	45 Gy
MGH[10]	0 out of 10	Optic neuropathy	50 Gy
Hearing Toxicities			
IRS II-III[32]	36 out of 213	High-frequency hearing loss	45 Gy
U of Iowa[31]	6 out of 8		
MSKCC[8]	—		
MGH[10]	0 out of 10		
Secondary Cancers			
IRS II-III[32]	4 out of 213		1.8 Gy
U of Iowa[31]	1 out of 17		
MSKCC[8]	2 out of 21		
MGH[10]	0 out of 10		

Abbreviations: ACTH, adrenocorticotropic hormone; GH, growth hormone; GnRH, gonadotrophin-releasing hormone; IRS, Intergroup Rhabdomyosarcoma Studies; MGH, Massachusetts General Hospital; MSKCC, Memorial Sloan Kettering Cancer Center; TMJ, temporomandibular joint; TSH, thyroid-stimulating hormone; U, university. *Data from* Refs. 8,10,31,32

increases to a 37% risk when cochlear doses are greater than 60 Gy. Radiation-induced hearing loss may be prevented by reducing the mean cochlear dose to less than 35 Gy and, if it occurs, may be treated with the use of hearing aids.

Secondary Cancers

Secondary cancers are among the most feared complications of radiotherapy in the pediatric age group. Between 3% and 5% of pediatric patients with cancer who survive 20 years or longer develop radiation-induced second malignancies.[56,57] The occurrence of a secondary neoplasm is dire because only 30% of children are curable.[58] After radiotherapy for soft tissue sarcomas, one report showed that the most common secondary tumors are bone sarcomas (n = 6), brain tumors (n = 3), leukemia (n = 2), and other sarcomas (n = 2).[58] Furthermore, in 13,136 pediatric cancer survivors, Bassal and colleagues[59] observed that 90% of secondary malignancies affecting the head and neck region occurred in patients who received prior head and neck radiotherapy.

With regard to radiation-induced cancers, the development of second malignancies depends on the radiation field and dose. Using a Nordic cancer registry, Svahn-Tapper and colleagues[60] showed that as little as 1 Gy was associated with a 1.8-fold increased risk of second malignancies, and this increased to a maximum risk of 18.3-fold for doses greater than 30 Gy. Furthermore, chemotherapy can additionally increase the risk of radiation-induced cancers from 2.3-fold to 4.3-fold. These secondary cancers tend to arise in the organs that reside within the radiation field, or reside immediately adjacent to the radiation fields. In 115 children who developed second solid malignancies, 12% of these cancers arose in the high-dose region; 66% of second cancers arose at the field edge, which received 50% of the radiation dose; and 22% arose more than 5 cm from the irradiated field (possibly caused by low-dose scattered radiation).[61] Furthermore, many of these second malignancies occurred in areas that received low radiation doses, because 31% of the secondary cancers arose in organs receiving less than 2.5 Gy.

SUMMARY

As long-term survival rates increase for pediatric cancers, so does the number of children at risk for long-term radiation morbidities. Irradiation of the head and neck region is associated with multiple radiation complications affecting many functions, including vision, hearing, eating, and growth. Furthermore, children receiving radiation

for head and neck cancers are at risk for developing second malignancies, which are associated with adverse outcomes. Approaches to reduce these risks of late radiation toxicities include using PBR and IGRT to more precisely target the cancer. In addition, these patients would benefit from more advances in medical interventions to prevent or mitigate radiation toxicities. Thus, improving the technical precision of radiation and medical management of radiation toxicities gives hope to the survivors of pediatric cancers.

REFERENCES

1. Murphy SL. Deaths: final data for 1998. Natl Vital Stat Rep 2000;48(11):1–105.
2. Jemal A, Tiwari RC, Murray T, et al. Cancer statistics, 2004. CA Cancer J Clin 2004;54(1):8–29.
3. DeSantis CE, Lin CC, Mariotto AB, et al. Cancer treatment and survivorship statistics, 2014. CA Cancer J Clin 2014;64(4):252–71.
4. Robison LL, Mertens AC, Boice JD, et al. Study design and cohort characteristics of the Childhood Cancer Survivor Study: a multi-institutional collaborative project. Med Pediatr Oncol 2002;38(4):229–39.
5. Albright JT, Topham AK, Reilly JS. Pediatric head and neck malignancies: US incidence and trends over 2 decades. Arch Otolaryngol Head Neck Surg 2002;128(6):655–9.
6. Lin C, Donaldson SS, Meza JL, et al. Effect of radiotherapy techniques (IMRT vs. 3D-CRT) on outcome in patients with intermediate-risk rhabdomyosarcoma enrolled in COG D9803–a report from the Children's Oncology Group. Int J Radiat Oncol Biol Phys 2012;82(5):1764–70.
7. Hein PA, Gladstone DJ, Bellerive MR, et al. Importance of protocol target definition on the ability to spare normal tissue: an IMRT and 3D-CRT planning comparison for intraorbital tumors. Int J Radiat Oncol Biol Phys 2005;62(5):1540–8.
8. McDonald MW, Esiashvili N, George BA, et al. Intensity-modulated radiotherapy with use of cone-down boost for pediatric head-and-neck rhabdomyosarcoma. Int J Radiat Oncol Biol Phys 2008;72(3):884–91.
9. Wolden SL, Wexler LH, Kraus DH, et al. Intensity modulated radiotherapy for head-and-neck rhabdomyosarcoma. Int J Radiat Oncol Biol Phys 2005;61(5):1432–8.
10. Fuss M, Hug EB, Schaefer RA, et al. Proton radiation therapy (PRT) for pediatric optic pathway gliomas: comparison with 3D planned conventional photons and a standard photon technique. Int J Radiat Oncol Biol Phys 1999;45(5):1117–26.
11. Yock T, Schneider R, Friedmann A, et al. Proton radiotherapy for orbital rhabdomyosarcoma: clinical

outcome and a dosimetric comparison with photons. Int J Radiat Oncol Biol Phys 2005;63(4):1161–8.

12. Ladra MM, Edgington SK, Mahajan A, et al. A dosimetric comparison of proton and intensity modulated radiation therapy in pediatric rhabdomyosarcoma patients enrolled on a prospective phase II proton study. Radiother Oncol 2014; 113(1):77–83.

13. Ladra MM, Szymonifka JD, Mahajan A, et al. Preliminary results of a phase II trial of proton radiotherapy for pediatric rhabdomyosarcoma. J Clin Oncol 2014; 32(33):3762–70.

14. De Ruysscher D, Mark Lodge M, Jones B, et al. Charged particles in radiotherapy: a 5-year update of a systematic review. Radiother Oncol 2012; 103(1):5–7.

15. Donaldson SS, Meza J, Breneman JC, et al. Results from the IRS-IV randomized trial of hyperfractionated radiotherapy in children with rhabdomyosarcoma–a report from the IRSG. Int J Radiat Oncol Biol Phys 2001;51(3):718–28.

16. Combs SE, Behnisch W, Kulozik AE, et al. Intensity modulated radiotherapy (IMRT) and fractionated stereotactic radiotherapy (FSRT) for children with head-and-neck-rhabdomyosarcoma. BMC Cancer 2007;7:177.

17. Miralbell R, Lomax A, Cella L, et al. Potential reduction of the incidence of radiation-induced second cancers by using proton beams in the treatment of pediatric tumors. Int J Radiat Oncol Biol Phys 2002;54(3):824–9.

18. Moteabbed M, Yock TI, Paganetti H. The risk of radiation-induced second cancers in the high to medium dose region: a comparison between passive and scanned proton therapy, IMRT and VMAT for pediatric patients with brain tumors. Phys Med Biol 2014;59(12):2883–99.

19. Chung CS, Yock TI, Nelson K, et al. Incidence of second malignancies among patients treated with proton versus photon radiation. Int J Radiat Oncol Biol Phys 2013;87(1):46–52.

20. Kozak KR, Adams J, Krejcarek SJ, et al. A dosimetric comparison of proton and intensity-modulated photon radiotherapy for pediatric parameningeal rhabdomyosarcomas. Int J Radiat Oncol Biol Phys 2009;74(1):179–86.

21. Allen AM, Pawlicki T, Dong L, et al. An evidence based review of proton beam therapy: the report of ASTRO's emerging technology committee. Radiother Oncol 2012;103(1):8–11.

22. Alcorn SR, Chen MJ, Claude L, et al. Practice patterns of photon and proton pediatric image guided radiation treatment: results from an International Pediatric Research consortium. Pract Radiat Oncol 2014;4(5):336–41.

23. Beltran C, Krasin MJ, Merchant TE. Inter- and intrafractional positional uncertainties in pediatric radiotherapy patients with brain and head and neck tumors. Int J Radiat Oncol Biol Phys 2011;79(4):1266–74.

24. Hensley ML, Schuchter LM, Lindley C, et al. American Society of Clinical Oncology clinical practice guidelines for the use of chemotherapy and radiotherapy protectants. J Clin Oncol 1999;17(10): 3333–55.

25. Anacak Y, Kamer S, Haydaroglu A. Daily subcutaneous amifostine administration during irradiation of pediatric head and neck cancers. Pediatr Blood Cancer 2007;48(5):579–81.

26. Marx RE, Johnson RP, Kline SN. Prevention of osteoradionecrosis: a randomized prospective clinical trial of hyperbaric oxygen versus penicillin. J Am Dent Assoc 1985;111(1):49–54.

27. Ashamalla HL, Thom SR, Goldwein JW. Hyperbaric oxygen therapy for the treatment of radiation-induced sequelae in children. The University of Pennsylvania experience. Cancer 1996;77(11):2407–12.

28. Moding EJ, Kastan MB, Kirsch DG. Strategies for optimizing the response of cancer and normal tissues to radiation. Nat Rev Drug Discov 2013;12(7): 526–42.

29. Holmqvist AS, Moell C, Hjorth L, et al. Increased health care utilization by survivors of childhood lymphoblastic leukemia is confined to those treated with cranial or total body irradiation: a case cohort study. BMC Cancer 2014;14:419.

30. Guyuron B, Dagys AP, Munro IR, et al. Effect of irradiation on facial growth: a 7- to 25-year follow-up. Ann Plast Surg 1983;11(5):423–7.

31. Kaste SC, Goodman P, Leisenring W, et al. Impact of radiation and chemotherapy on risk of dental abnormalities: a report from the Childhood Cancer Survivor Study. Cancer 2009;115(24):5817–27.

32. Paulino AC, Simon JH, Zhen W, et al. Long-term effects in children treated with radiotherapy for head and neck rhabdomyosarcoma. Int J Radiat Oncol Biol Phys 2000;48(5):1489–95.

33. Raney RB, Asmar L, Vassilopoulou-Sellin R, et al. Late complications of therapy in 213 children with localized, nonorbital soft-tissue sarcoma of the head and neck: a descriptive report from the Intergroup Rhabdomyosarcoma Studies (IRS)-II and -III. IRS Group of the Children's Cancer Group and the Pediatric Oncology Group. Med Pediatr Oncol 1999;33(4):362–71.

34. Cubukcu CE, Sevinir B, Ercan I. Disturbed dental development of permanent teeth in children with solid tumors and lymphomas. Pediatr Blood Cancer 2012;58(1):80–4.

35. Sonis AL, Tarbell N, Valachovic RW, et al. Dentofacial development in long-term survivors of acute lymphoblastic leukemia. A comparison of three treatment modalities. Cancer 1990;66(12):2645–52.

36. Holtta P, Alaluusua S, Saarinen-Pihkala UM, et al. Long-term adverse effects on dentition in children

with poor-risk neuroblastoma treated with high-dose chemotherapy and autologous stem cell transplantation with or without total body irradiation. Bone Marrow Transplant 2002;29(2):121–7.

37. Nasman M, Bjork O, Soderhall S, et al. Disturbances in the oral cavity in pediatric long-term survivors after different forms of antineoplastic therapy. Pediatr Dent 1994;16(3):217–23.

38. Meazza C, Ferrari A, Casanova M, et al. Evolving treatment strategies for parameningeal rhabdomyosarcoma: the experience of the Istituto Nazionale Tumori of Milan. Head Neck 2005;27(1):49–57.

39. Bolling T, Weege J, Eich HT, et al. Acute and late side effects to salivary glands and oral mucosa after head and neck radiotherapy in children and adolescents. Results of the "Registry for the Evaluation of Side Effects after Radiotherapy in Childhood and Adolescence". Head Neck 2015;37(8): 1137–41.

40. Deasy JO, Moiseenko V, Marks L, et al. Radiotherapy dose-volume effects on salivary gland function. Int J Radiat Oncol Biol Phys 2010;76(3 Suppl I):S58–63.

41. Krasin MJ, Xiong X, Wu S, et al. The effects of external beam irradiation on the growth of flat bones in children: modeling a dose-volume effect. Int J Radiat Oncol Biol Phys 2005;62(5):1458–63.

42. Mercado CE, Little SB, Mazewski C, et al. Mandibular condyle erosion and sclerosis in pediatric patients treated with radiotherapy to the head and neck region. Pediatr Blood Cancer 2014;61(8):1479–80.

43. Gevorgyan A, La Scala GC, Neligan PC, et al. Radiation-induced craniofacial bone growth disturbances. J Craniofac Surg 2007;18(5):1001–7.

44. Pertschuk MJ, Whitaker LA. Psychosocial adjustment and craniofacial malformations in childhood. Plast Reconstr Surg 1985;75(2):177–84.

45. Pertschuk MJ, Whitaker LA. Psychosocial outcome of craniofacial surgery in children. Plast Reconstr Surg 1988;82(5):741–6.

46. Pope AW, Snyder HT. Psychosocial adjustment in children and adolescents with a craniofacial anomaly: age and sex patterns. Cleft Palate Craniofac J 2005;42(4):349–54.

47. Cohen SR, Bartlett SP, Whitaker LA. Reconstruction of late craniofacial deformities after irradiation of the head and face during childhood. Plast Reconstr Surg 1990;86(2):229–37.

48. Jackson IT, Carls F, Bush K, et al. Assessment and treatment of facial deformity resulting from radiation to the orbital area in childhood. Plast Reconstr Surg 1996;98(7):1169–79 [discussion: 1180–1].

49. Gurlek A, Miller MJ, Amin AA, et al. Reconstruction c complex radiation-induced injuries using free-tissue transfer. J Reconstr Microsurg 1998;14(5):337–40.

50. Bhandare N, Kennedy L, Malyapa RS, et al. Hypopi tuitarism after radiotherapy for extracranial head and neck cancers in pediatric patients. Am J Clin Onco 2008;31(6):567–72.

51. Brauner R, Czernichow P, Rappaport R. Greate susceptibility to hypothalamopituitary irradiation ir younger children with acute lymphoblastic leukemia J Pediatr 1986;108(2):332.

52. Shalet SM. Radiation and pituitary dysfunction N Engl J Med 1993;328(2):131–3.

53. Jeganathan VS, Wirth A, MacManus MP. Ocula risks from orbital and periorbital radiation therapy a critical review. Int J Radiat Oncol Biol Phys 2011 79(3):650–9.

54. Hoehn ME, Irshad F, Kerr NC, et al. Outcomes afte cataract extraction in young children with radiation induced cataracts and retinoblastoma. J AAPOS 2010;14(3):232–4.

55. Hua C, Bass JK, Khan R, et al. Hearing loss afte radiotherapy for pediatric brain tumors: effect o cochlear dose. Int J Radiat Oncol Biol Phys 2008 72(3):892–9.

56. Gold DG, Neglia JP, Potish RA, et al. Second neo plasms following megavoltage radiation for pediatric tumors. Cancer 2004;100(1):212–3.

57. Neglia JP, Friedman DL, Yasui Y, et al. Second malignant neoplasms in five-year survivors of childhood cancer: childhood cancer survivor study J Natl Cancer Inst 2001;93(8):618–29.

58. Rich DC, Corpron CA, Smith MB, et al. Second malignant neoplasms in children after treatment o soft tissue sarcoma. J Pediatr Surg 1997;32(2) 369–72.

59. Bassal M, Mertens AC, Taylor L, et al. Risk o selected subsequent carcinomas in survivors o childhood cancer: a report from the Childhood Cancer Survivor Study. J Clin Oncol 2006;24(3) 476–83.

60. Svahn-Tapper G, Garwicz S, Anderson H, et al. Radiation dose and relapse are predictors for development of second malignant solid tumors after cance in childhood and adolescence: a population-based case-control study in the five Nordic countries Acta Oncol 2006;45(4):438–48.

61. Diallo I, Haddy N, Adjadj E, et al. Frequency distribution of second solid cancer locations in relation to the irradiated volume among 115 patients treated for childhood cancer. Int J Radiat Onco Biol Phys 2009;74(3):876–83.

Chemotherapy in Children with Head and Neck Cancers
Perspectives and Review of Current Therapies

Daniel K. Choi, MD, MS*, Mary Lou Schmidt, MD

KEYWORDS

- Chemotherapy • Pediatric cancer • Lymphoma • Retinoblastoma • Rhabdomyosarcoma
- Neuroblastoma

KEY POINTS

- The head and neck are common sites for cancers in children and young adults; although usually from metastatic disease, several pediatric malignancies originate in various head and neck structures.
- Non-Hodgkin and Hodgkin lymphoma comprise the most common head and neck malignancies seen in children and young adults; other important malignancies include rhabdomyosarcoma, neuroblastoma, and Langerhans cell histiocytosis.
- Chemotherapy is often required to treat head and neck malignancies in children and young adults, and is associated with acute toxicities, late effects, and potential additional morbidity when combined with radiation and/or surgical therapies.
- Survival rates are favorable for many malignancies of the head and neck in children and young adults.
- As more children and young adults survive treatment for their head and neck malignancies, providers must be vigilant in monitoring for potential late effects of therapy, as well as ensuring proper transitioning of their patients to adult care.

INTRODUCTION

Cancers of the head and neck constitute approximately 12% of all cancers in children ages 1 to 15 years in the United States.[1] Specific incidence estimates outside the United States are not widely reported, although Gosepath and colleagues[2] reported the incidence of head and neck cancers in a large cohort of German children to be 4.48 per 100,000. Both these estimates specifically excluded primary brain and spinal tumors, which are also omitted for the purposes of this review. The most common malignancies in children presenting in the head and neck are shown in **Fig. 1**. In their analysis of the Surveillance, Epidemiology, and End Results (SEER) registry from 1973 to 1996, Albright and colleagues[1] found that lymphomas, neural tumors, thyroid malignancies, and soft tissue sarcomas comprised greater than 80% of the 3050 head and neck tumors diagnosed in children during that

Financial Disclosures: The authors have nothing to disclose.

Division of Pediatric Hematology/Oncology, Department of Pediatrics, University of Illinois at Chicago College of Medicine, 840 South Wood Street, MC 856, Chicago, IL 60612, USA

* Corresponding author.

E-mail address: dkchoi@uic.edu

Oral Maxillofacial Surg Clin N Am 28 (2016) 127–138

http://dx.doi.org/10.1016/j.coms.2015.08.004

1042-3699/16/$ – see front matter © 2016 Elsevier Inc. All rights reserved.

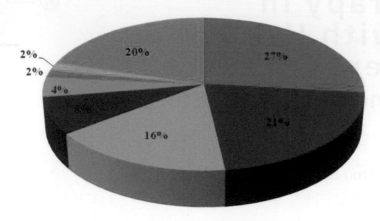

Fig. 1. Common pediatric malignancies of the head and neck (*Data from* Albright JT, Topham AK, Reilly JS. Pediatric head and neck malignancies: US incidence and trends over 2 decades. Arch Otolaryngol Head Neck Surg 2002;128(6):655–9.)

■ Lymphoma (Hodgkin's and Non-Hodgkin's)   ■ Thyroid Carcinoma

■ Retinoblastoma   ■ Rhabdomyosarcoma

■ Non-Rhabomyosarcoma Soft Tissue Sarcomas   ■ Neuroblastoma

■ Squamos Cell Carcinoma   ■ Other

period. Incidence estimates are complicated by overlapping definitions of pediatric cancers that are exclusive to the head and neck versus the more common malignancies that can originate at other sites, including the head and neck (eg, rhabdomyosarcoma). Based on an analysis of the SEER registry from 1973 to 2008 by Cesmebasi and colleagues,[3] excluding common malignancies that can originate at other sites, the incidence of cancers in children originating exclusively in the head and neck region was approximately 0.25 per 100,000. The analysis noted the 5 most common anatomic sites involved, in order of frequency, were (1) salivary glands; (2) nasopharynx; (3) nose, nasal cavity, and middle ear; (4) gum and other mouth; and (5) tongue, and almost all were of squamous cell carcinoma (SCC) histology.

The age of a child at which they present with a head and neck malignancy is an important consideration. For example, malignancies presenting in the head and neck of children age birth to 5 years old will commonly include neuroblastoma or retinoblastoma, which are exceedingly rare in older children. In adolescents and young adults (AYAs), head and neck malignancies are more likely to be lymphomas, soft tissue sarcomas, and other common adult cancers, such as SCC. Determining prognosis and appropriate treatments for young patients with head and neck malignancies requires risk stratification. Patient characteristics included in risk stratification commonly include age, anatomic site(s) involved, extent of surgical resection, presence of metastatic disease, molecular/cytogenetic features of the malignancy, histologic type/differentiation of the malignancy, and responsiveness to therapy.

On confirmation of the diagnosis, many cancers of the head and neck will require close coordination among providers regarding the timing of chemotherapy and administration of concurrent therapies. In many cases, after a biopsy or primary resection of a head and neck tumor, patients will require time for postoperative wound healing. In this instance, initiation of chemotherapy may be delayed so as to avoid poor wound healing due to general immune suppression, specifically due to chemotherapy's effect on neutrophil number and function. In addition, several malignancies of the head and neck often require radiation therapy. In managing the side effects of radiation to the head and neck, providers need to be acutely aware that many chemotherapeutic agents can impair healing at the irradiated site, and even potentiate the toxic effects of radiation (eg, doxorubicin, actinomycin-D). Knowledge of issues related to the administration of chemotherapy in various head and neck malignancies in children is critical to allow practitioners to better manage their patients while undergoing these crucial therapies. A summary of common chemotherapeutic agents used in treating pediatric malignancies of the head and neck is shown in **Table 1**.

CANCERS OF THE HEAD AND NECK
Lymphoma

Lymphoma, composed of Hodgkin lymphoma (HL) and non-Hodgkin lymphoma (NHL), is the third most common malignancy diagnosed in children in the United States (after acute leukemia and primary brain tumors). Annually, there are approximately 1700 new cases of lymphoma diagnosed

Table 1
Chemotherapeutic agents used in the treatment of pediatric head and neck cancers

Chemotherapy Agent	Malignancies Treated	Acute Toxicity(s)	Potential Late Effect[19]
Vincristine	LL, RMS, HL, NHL, NB, RB	Peripheral neuropathy, constipation, SIADH	Chronic peripheral neuropathy, Raynaud syndrome
Vinblastine	LCH	Myelosuppression	—
Cyclophosphamide	LL, RMS, HL, NHL, NB	Hemorrhagic cystitis, myelosuppression	Infertility, t-AML, bladder carcinoma
Iphosphamide	RMS[a]	Neurotoxicity, electrolyte loss/Fanconi syndrome	Nephrotoxicity
Doxorubicin	LL, RMS, HL, NHL, NB	Cardiomyopathy, myelosuppression, liver injury, radiation recall	Cardiomyopathy, arrhythmias, early atherosclerosis, t-AML
Daunorubicin	LL		
Actinomycin-D	RMS		—
Etoposide	HL, RMS,[a] NB, RB	Myelosuppression	t-AML
Bleomycin	HL	Rash, allergic reactions	Pulmonary fibrosis
Cisplatin	NB, SCC	Severe nausea/vomiting, myelosuppression, nephrotoxicity	Sensorineural hearing loss, neuropathy, nephrotoxicity
Carboplatin	NB,[b] RB		
Topotecan	NB[a]	Diarrhea	—
Irinotecan	RMS[a]		
Prednisone	LL, NHL, HL, LCH	Cushingoid features, emotional labiality, hyperglycemia	Osteopenia, avascular necrosis of the hip, growth disturbances, cataracts
Dexamethasone	LL		
Methotrexate	LL, NHL[c]	Myelosuppression, neurotoxicity (when given intrathecally), nephrotoxicity	Neurocognitive deficits
Cytarabine	LL, NHL[c]	Fever, myelosuppression, rash	Neurocognitive deficits
L-Asparaginase	LL	Allergic reaction/anaphylaxis, coagulopathy, pancreatitis	—
Mercaptopurine	LL	Myelosuppression, liver injury	—
Thioguanine	LL	Myelosuppression, liver injury	—

Abbreviations: HL, Hodgkin lymphoma; LCH, Langerhans cell histiocytosis; NB, neuroblastoma; RB, retinoblastoma; RMS, rhabdomyosarcoma; SIADH, syndrome of inappropriate anti-diuretic hormone; t-AML, therapy-related acute myelogenous leukemia.
[a] Only in high-risk disease.
[b] Only in intermediate-risk disease.
[c] Only NHL risk groups B and C.
Data from Children's Oncology Group. Long-term follow-up guidelines for survivors of childhood, adolescent and young adult cancers, version 4.0. Monrovia, CA: Children's Oncology Group 2013.

n children and AYAs in the United States.[4] In infants and young children, NHL is much more common, with more than 600 new patients ages birth to 14 years diagnosed annually.[5] In contrast, HL is less common in younger children, but is the most common malignancy diagnosed in children older than 15 years, with more than 800 patients ages 15 to 18 years diagnosed annually.[5] Although lymphomas most commonly arise from nodal sites in the head and neck, extranodal involvement can occur in the mucosa of the paranasal sinuses, oral mucosa, and salivary glands.[6] In multiple series, lymphomas accounted for the single largest proportion of cancers in the head and neck in children, from 27% to 55%.[1,7–9] Specific populations of pediatric patients are also at increased risk for the development of lymphomas, including those with either acquired or congenital immunodeficiencies, and after solid organ transplantation (posttransplant lymphoproliferative disorder).

NHLs make up approximately 60% of all childhood lymphomas, presenting in the head and neck in approximately 10% of cases in children.[7] As noted previously, NHL is traditionally seen in younger children, often presenting as painless lymphadenopathy. The time course for the enlargement of involved lymph nodes in NHL exists on a spectrum, from gradual enlargement over several months, to rapid growth in a matter of days to weeks. Constitutional symptoms can be seen but are more traditionally associated with HL "B" symptoms, defined as persistent fevers for longer than 3 days, 10% or greater weight loss in the previous 6 months, and drenching night sweats. Although the 2008 World Health Organization classification system has recognized more than 100 unique subtypes of lymphomas,[10] most subtypes seen in children include Burkitt lymphoma (BL), lymphoblastic lymphoma (LL), diffuse large B-cell lymphoma (DLBCL), and anaplastic large cell lymphoma (ALCL). In general, the type and duration of chemotherapy for NHL is determined by the stage of disease, response to initial therapy, and specific molecular and cytogenetic features. The St Jude/Murphy staging and risk stratification criteria for NHL used by pediatric oncologists is shown in **Table 2**.[11,12] An important adjunct to establishing the stage of the NHL often includes a bone marrow biopsy and cerebrospinal fluid (CSF) examination before initiating any systemic treatments, including corticosteroids.

BL and DLBCL represent the two most common B-cell lymphomas in children, and are treated with similar regimens of chemotherapy. BL is more common in younger children, with a median age of presentation of 8.4 years compared with 11.4 years for DLBCL.[13] The incidence of these subtypes of NHL also depends on gender, with BL being more common in boys (4.5:1.0 compared with an equal incidence of DLBCL in boys versus girls.[13]

BL is the most common NHL, constituting approximately 25% of all NHLs seen in children BL most commonly presents as a rapidly proliferating abdominal or mediastinal mass. When presenting as isolated lymphadenopathy, BL can involve the lymph nodes of the head and neck in up to 50% of cases.[14] BL can also involve the bone marrow and central nervous system (CNS) In the endemic form of BL seen in equatorial Africa large masses of the jaw and periorbital region are common, and are strongly associated with concurrent Epstein-Barr virus (EBV) infection. In contrast, DLBCL more typically presents as localized disease, with head and neck structures more likely to be secondary sites of disease extension from the mediastinum, the most common site of presentation in DLBCL. Unlike BL, the bone marrow and CNS are rarely involved in DLBCL.[15]

There are several combinations of chemotherapy that have proven effective against BL DLBCL. Depending on stage, a common treatment protocol for BL and DLBCL involves the administration of cyclophosphamide, Oncovin (vincristine), prednisone, and Adriamycin (doxorubicin) ± methotrexate. This regimen, often referred to as COPAD-M, is administered for up to 3 cycles, and can be followed with a combination of

Table 2
St Jude/Murphy staging and risk stratification criteria for non-Hodgkin lymphoma

Stage	Sites
I	Single nodal or extranodal tumor excluding the mediastinum and abdomen
II	a. Single extranodal tumor with regional node involvement, or b. Two or more nodal areas on the same side of the diaphragm, or c. Two extranodal tumors on the same side of the diaphragm (with or without regional node involvement) d. Primary gastrointestinal tract tumor that is resectable
III	a. Two extranodal tumors on opposite sides of the diaphragm b. Two or more nodal areas above and below the diaphragm, or c. Any intrathoracic disease (lung, pleura, mediastinum, and thymic), or d. All extensive, primary intra-abdominal disease, or e. All paraspinal or epidural disease (regardless of other tumor sites)
IV	Bone marrow and/or central nervous system (CNS) involvement
	Risk Group Stratification A. Completely resected stage I or completely resected abdominal stage II lesions B. All nonresected tumors stages I–IV (no CNS disease, bone marrow <25% blasts) C. Any CNS disease and/or bone marrow involvement ≥25% blasts

Adapted from Murphy SB. Classification, staging and end results of treatment of childhood non-Hodgkin's lymphomas dissimilarities from lymphomas in adults. Semin Oncol 1980;7(3):332–9; and Patte C, Auperin A, Gerrard M, et al. Results of the randomized international FAB/LMB96 trial for intermediate risk B-cell non-Hodgkin lymphoma in children and adolescents: it is possible to reduce treatment for the early responding patients. Blood 2007;109(7):2773–80.

cyclophosphamide, cytarabine, and methotrexate regimen abbreviated CYM) for an additional 2 cycles. Stage and risk group will determine the number of cycles of chemotherapy given, with total treatment duration lasting from 2 to 6 months. This treatment regimen was evaluated by the French-American-British (FAB)/LMB96 trial, enrolling more than 650 children with BL and DLBCL. The LMB96 trial demonstrated that the most common associated toxicities with COPAD-M included (1) moderate to severe oropharyngeal stomatitis (mucositis) and (2) severe infection, occurring in greater than 20% and 8% of patients, respectively.[12] The study reported that a reduction in cyclophosphamide dose could significantly reduce the frequency of these toxicities without affecting survival rates. Indeed, the survival rates were excellent for all patients, with a 4-year event-free survival (EFS) of 93.4% and 90.9% (relative risk = 1.3, P = .40) in the groups with full and half doses of cyclophosphamide, respectively.[12]

Unlike the B-cell lymphomas of BL and DLBCL, LL is more likely a malignancy of T cells, and is treated differently. Overall, LL constitutes approximately 20% of all childhood NHLs.[13] The T-cell phenotype constitutes 75% of all LLs diagnosed in children.[16] T-cell LL (T-LL) in children often presents as a mediastinal mass, sometimes with an associated pleural effusion. T-LL in the head and neck is usually lymphadenopathy due to extension from a primary mediastinal mass, although other areas, such as the thyroid, can be affected at presentation.[17] Treatment of T-LL has evolved over the years, due in large part to the realization that T-LL is genetically more similar to T-acute lymphoblastic leukemia (T-ALL) than other lymphomas. Indeed, it is now accepted that T-ALL and T-LL exist as a spectrum of the same disease, with T-ALL being defined as greater than 25% lymphoblasts present in the bone marrow at diagnosis.

Treatment of T-LL is now identical to that given for children with T-ALL. The mainstay of therapy is intensive chemotherapy with 9 to 11 chemotherapeutic agents over 8 to 10 months followed by 2 years of monthly outpatient maintenance therapy. CNS prophylaxis with intrathecal chemotherapy ± cranial irradiation is included throughout treatment. Therapy is delivered for a total of 2.5 years in girls, and 3.5 years in boys to achieve equivalent survival rates. Effects of the common chemotherapeutic agents used to treat T-LL are shown in **Table 1**. Using leukemia-based treatment protocols for T-LL, 5-year EFS is now 90%.[18] It is important to note that given the duration of treatment, there are notable late effects associated with intensive T-LL treatment, which are also outlined in **Table 1**.[19]

Similar to T-LL, ALCL is a T-cell lymphoma, specifically of mature T cells. Collectively, ALCL constitutes 10% of all NHLs seen in children, and has shown a male predominance.[13,20] ALCL has a heterogeneous presentation, making the diagnosis difficult unless there is a high index of suspicion by practitioners. Unique aspects of ALCL include the frequent presence of constitutional symptoms, such as fever (75%), extranodal involvement, and bony involvement (including the skull).[20,21] ALCL is also unique among NHLs in its presentation in the skin (cutaneous ALCL), seen in up to 20% of patients.[20] The current recommended therapy for patients with ALCL is chemotherapy with doxorubicin, prednisone, and vincristine (abbreviated APO) given over 52 weeks. This regimen is overall well tolerated, and can be given as an outpatient. However, several trials have demonstrated alternative regimens involving shorter, more-intensive chemotherapy can achieve similar outcomes, but with notable hematologic toxicities (primarily significant neutropenia).[22–24]

Overall outcomes for children with ALCL treated with chemotherapy remain unsatisfactory, with 5-year EFS of only 65% to 72%.[22–24] In addition, up to 25% of patients will have progression while on therapy, necessitating hematopoietic stem cell transplantation (HSCT). However, increasing knowledge of the molecular features of ALCL has paved the way for new investigational agents that could improve overall survival (OS). The ALCL kinase (Alk) fusion protein is believed to contribute to the pathogenesis of ALCL. Significant differences in OS have been demonstrated in Alk-positive versus Alk-negative lymphomas, 71% versus 15% (P<.007), respectively.[20] In addition, ALCL often expresses CD30 on its cell surface. The Children's Oncology Group (COG), a research consortium of more than 200 institutions providing pediatric cancer care, is currently examining the role of specific targeted therapies, brentuximab vedotin (anti-CD30 antibody) versus crizotinib (an Alk tyrosine kinase inhibitor) in addition to standard chemotherapy in a head-to-head Phase II trial.

HL is the most common malignancy diagnosed in AYAs ages15 to 25 years, and constitutes 40% of all lymphomas diagnosed in children and AYAs. HL typically presents as a painless cervical or supraclavicular lymph node. Mediastinal lymphadenopathy can lead to significant cough, orthopnea, and superior vena cava syndrome. Unlike NHL, constitutional "B" symptoms in HL are common in up to 25% of patients, and are of prognostic significance.[25] HL spreads contiguously from one lymph node to the next, and extranodal involvement other than the spleen is rare except in patients with an underlying immunodeficiency, such as human immunodeficiency virus.[26] The staging and risk stratification for HL are shown in **Table 3**.[27]

The mainstay of therapy for patients with HL remains chemotherapy and radiation. Chemotherapy for HL typically involves administering cyclophosphamide, vincristine, prednisone, and procarbazine (abbreviated COPP) or Adriamycin, bleomycin, vincristine, etoposide, prednisone, and cyclophosphamide (abbreviated ABVE-PC). There are several variations to these regimens based on risk stratification, such as the omission of cyclophosphamide, bleomycin, and etoposide from ABVE-PC in low-risk disease.[28] The most common side effect of this combination of agents is profound myelosuppression, and supportive care with granulocyte colony-stimulating factor (G-CSF) is indicated to hasten blood count recovery and reduce infection risks. Therapy duration is generally 3 to 6 months depending on the number of cycles indicated, with response to therapy being a key indicator of OS.[29] Unlike most NHLs, radiation therapy is indicated in the treatment of HL, although there is evidence that it can be omitted in certain patients with low-risk HL.[28,30,31] Survival rates for patients with HL consistently surpass 90%.[28–31] However, there are significant late effects associated with the treatment of HL, such as cardiovascular disease, infertility, and secondary malignancies. Research efforts to minimize chemotherapy and radiation exposure without compromising survival outcomes are ongoing.

Sarcomas

Pediatric soft tissue sarcomas are subdivided into the common rhabdomyosarcoma (RMS) and a heterogeneous group of benign and malignant tumors called nonrhabdomyosarcoma soft tissue sarcomas (NRSTS). Collectively, soft tissue sarcomas represent 7% of all pediatric malignancies and RMS alone accounts for 3% of all malignancies in children.[4] There are 3 histologic subtypes of RMS, embryonal, alveolar, and mixed undifferentiated, making up 70%, 20%, and 10% of cases, respectively. RMS is more likely in younger children, with more than 50% of cases diagnosed in children younger than 10 years.[4]

The head and neck is a common site of presentation for RMS, occurring in up to 35% of cases.[33] RMS in the head and neck includes the orbit, parameninges (nasopharynx/nasal cavity, the middle ear, the paranasal sinuses, and infratemporal fossa/pterygopalatine space), and nonparameninges in 26%, 44%, and 30% of patients, respectively.[33] Location within the head and neck is also important in RMS risk stratification, which is determined by a combination of stage (anatomic location) and group (surgical), as shown in **Table 4**.[3] RMS of the orbit and nonparameninges are considered stage I favorable sites, whereas the parameningeal sites are stages 2 to 4 and are unfavorable sites. Metastatic disease (stage IV group 4), usually to the lungs and bone marrow, is seen in 16% of RMS at presentation.[35]

Treatment for RMS involves a combination of chemotherapy and local control of residual disease

---

Table 3
Ann Arbor staging system and risk stratification for Hodgkin lymphoma

Stage	Sites	Risk Group
I	Single node region (I) or single extranodal organ or site (I_E).	Low: IA, no bulk Intermediate: IA + bulk, I_EA/B
II	Two or more node regions on the same side of the diaphragm (II) or 1 node region and localized extranodal site on the same side of the diaphragm (II_E).	Low: IIA, no bulk Intermediate: IIA + bulk, II_EA, IIB
III	Node regions are involved on both sides of the diaphragm (III) and may include a localized extranodal site (III_E), the spleen (III_S), or both (III_{SE}).	Intermediate: IIIA High: IIIB
IV	Diffuse/disseminated involvement of more than 1 extranodal site.	Intermediate: IVA High: IVB

Additional Definitions: A, no symptoms; B, symptoms of persistent fevers for more than 3 days, 10% or greater weight loss in the previous 6 months and drenching night sweats.

Bulk Disease: (1) Mediastinal mass: tumor greater than 1/3 thoracic diameter on chest radiograph, (2) nonmediastinal nodal aggregate greater than 6 cm in the longest transverse diameter, or (3) macroscopic splenic nodules: focal defects on computed tomography, PET, or MRI.

From Carbone PP, Kaplan HS, Musshoff K, et al. Report of the Committee on Hodgkin's disease staging classification. Cancer Res 1971;31(11):1861.

Table 4
Risk stratification in pediatric rhabdomyosarcoma

Risk Group	Proportion of Cases	Sites
Low	35%	Stage I, Group I, II, III ERMS (favorable site and histology, localized) Stage II/III, Group I, II (unfavorable site, favorable histology, grossly resected)
Intermediate	50%	All localized ARMS (unfavorable histology) Stage II/III, Group III ERMS (unfavorable site, favorable histology, gross residual)
High	15%	Metastatic disease

Staging (Anatomic Location): Stage I, orbit, nonparameningeal head and neck, non–bladder/prostate genitourinary, biliary tract; Stage II, parameningeal, bladder/prostate, extremity, any other site, <5 cm and/or no regional nodal involvement; Stage III, parameningeal, bladder/prostate, extremity, any other site, ≥5 cm and/or regional nodal involvement; Stage IV, metastatic disease.

Group (Surgical): Group I, localized disease, completely resected; Group II, gross total resection, microscopic residual disease; Group III, incomplete resection with gross residual disease; Group IV, metastatic disease.

Abbreviations: ARMS, alveolar rhabdomyosarcoma; ERMS, embryonal rhabdomyosarcoma.

Adapted from Breneman JC, Lyden E, Pappo AS, et al. Prognostic factors and clinical outcomes in children and adolescents with metastatic rhabdomyosarcoma—a report from the Intergroup Rhabdomyosarcoma Study IV. J Clin Oncol 2003;21(1):78.

with surgery (when feasible) and/or radiation. Based on the current COG risk stratification system, patients will receive vincristine, actinomycin-D, and cyclophosphamide (abbreviated VDC) for 24 or 42 weeks for low-risk and intermediate-risk disease. Chemotherapy is administered weekly, with more intensive chemotherapy required every 2 to 3 weeks with G-CSF support to minimize delays in therapy and decrease infection risks. For high-risk disease, irinotecan, iphosphamide, and etoposide are added to VDC, various combinations of which are given over 1 year. This intensive regimen, often referred to as interval compression chemotherapy, is associated with notable myelosuppression and gastrointestinal toxicities. Despite the myelosuppressive effects, multiple studies in patients with RMS and Ewing sarcoma have demonstrated that interval compression chemotherapy can be delivered safely, thereby maximizing early exposure of the tumor to these effective combinations.[36]

In all risk groups, chemotherapy is continued when radiation therapy is initiated (usually 6–20 weeks after starting therapy). The exception to this schedule occurs in parameningeal RMS with intracranial extension, where radiation is administered at the start of therapy. In addition, actinomycin-D can act as a radiation sensitizer, and is therefore omitted during cycles that overlap with radiation therapy to minimize toxicity.

In their analysis of head and neck RMS in the SEER registry, Turner and Richmon[33] noted that the 5-year survival rates for patients diagnosed from 1973 to 2007 was 62.8%. Based on its location as a favorable site, orbital RMS has higher OS rates of greater than 90%. Depending on risk group, parameningeal RMS has more variable OS rates of 32% to 82%.[37–39] In addition, OS rates in RMS must be cautiously interpreted, as important prognostic factors of age, favorable versus unfavorable site, size of the tumor, extent of local control, and histologic subtype all contribute significantly to OS. Indeed, several reports have consistently demonstrated worse outcomes for patients with alveolar compared with embryonal RMS, with overall survival of 48% to 66% versus 73% to 83%, respectively.[40,41] OS for metastatic RMS with intensive therapy remains poor at 39%,[34] and therefore new effective agents and regimens are urgently needed to improve outcomes for this group of patients.

Neuroblastoma

Neuroblastoma (NB) is the most common extracranial solid tumor in children, and the most common solid tumor in children younger than 1 year.[5] Approximately 700 children are diagnosed annually with NB, with a vast majority of these children diagnosed by age 5.[4,5] NB is a tumor of neural crest cells, which can migrate anywhere along the neuraxis. Therefore, NB can have a heterogeneous clinical presentation, with the adrenal gland being the most common site of involvement and presenting as an abdominal mass. NB presenting in the head and neck is more often a manifestation of metastatic disease, as most patients present with advanced stage disease. Metastatic NB to the head and neck can manifest as painless cervical lymphadenopathy, periorbital ecchymosis ("raccoon eyes"), proptosis, and Horner syndrome.[42] Primary NB of the head and neck region is rare, accounting for only 2% to 5% of all cases.[43,44] Presentations can occur as cervical lymphadenopathy, but also can be primary tumors of the oropharynx and nasopharynx (esthioneuroblastoma, seen more commonly in AYAs). As head and neck sites are more likely metastatic foci and not primary disease, a thorough investigation for the extent of disease must be undertaken. The diagnostic workup for NB includes biopsy of the primary tumor, computed tomography of the neck/chest/abdomen/pelvis, urine catecholamines, metaiodobenzylguanidine (mIBG) scan and bone marrow biopsy.

Treatment for NB is highly dependent on risk stratification, which is determined by age, image-defined risk factors, favorable versus unfavorable histology, and molecular features (DNA ploidy, MYCN gene amplified vs nonamplified). Each of these risk factors has proven to be important in determining the overall prognosis for a child with NB.[45] Based on these risk factors, treatment can vary from observation and/or surgery in low-risk patients, 4 to 8 cycles of moderate-dose chemotherapy and surgery in intermediate-risk patients, to intensive chemotherapy, surgery, radiation, autologous HSCT, and maintenance therapy with targeted immune therapies plus retinoic acid in high-risk patients. The chemotherapy agents used in the treatment of NB are extensive, and are summarized as part of **Table 1**. In addition to the highly myelosuppressive effects of these regimens, particular emphasis needs to be placed on specific agents. Treatment of high-risk NB involves high cumulative doses of anthracyclines, with a concomitant increased risk of cardiotoxic effects. NB treatments also rely on the use of platinum agents, and higher cumulative doses are associated with an increased risk of high-frequency hearing loss and nephrotoxicity. Finally, patients with high-risk NB undergo autologous HSCT, and its involved chemotherapy regimens are associated with profound myelosuppression, infections, and sinusoidal obstructive syndrome (from busulfan).

Due to the heterogeneity of disease in NB, OS depends on a patient's risk stratification. OS for patients with low-risk and intermediate-risk disease remains strong at 93% to 98% depending on various clinical and biological features.[46] However, despite high-dose chemotherapy, surgery, radiation, HSCT, and immune-based therapies, the results for high-risk NB continue to be disappointing. The most recently reported data from the COG show a 2-year survival rate of only 30% to 40%.[42,47] OS data specifically for head and neck primary NB is limited due to the relative paucity of cases. However, primary head and neck NB may be more amenable to successful treatment with surgery and chemotherapy due to their lower overall stage and lack of MYCN amplification.[44] Indeed, OS for neck NB when compared with an adrenal primary tumor had a hazard ratio of 0.54 (95% confidence interval 0.31–0.94, P<.029) corresponding with several small case series reporting OS rates of greater than 90%.[44,48,49]

Other Notable Pediatric Head and Neck Malignancies

There are several other notable malignancies of the head and neck seen in children and AYAs that often require treatment with chemotherapy. To begin with, retinoblastoma (RB) is a uniquely pediatric malignancy, and is the most common ocular tumor in children. Annually more than 250 children, usually by age 5, are diagnosed with RB in the United States.[50] Most children present with isolated leukocoria, and are often referred directly to an ophthalmologist. Children possessing a germline mutation in the Rb tumor suppressor gene will have bilateral disease, although the extent of disease can vary between each eye. Extraorbital RB is indicative of advanced disease and can present with symptoms including proptosis, pain, and even loss of vision. Although more common internationally, extraorbital disease is rare in the United States, occurring in fewer than 10% of patients.[51] Staging is critical in the diagnosis of RB, as treatment involves a balance between the preservation of vision and limiting the extent of the disease within the affected eye(s). Current treatments include systemic chemotherapy, intraocular chemotherapy, cryosurgery, and laser surgery, radiation, and when necessary, enucleation of the affected eye. The common chemotherapeutic agents used to treat RB and their associated toxicities are summarized as part of **Table 1**. OS rates for ocular RB remain positive, with conventional therapy yielding greater than 95% survival in children.[50]

Langerhans cell histiocytosis (LCH) is a histiocytic disorder with a variable clinical presentation. The exact incidence of LCH in children is unknown, as the disease is often underrecognized or misdiagnosed. Recent estimates of the incidence of LCH in children are 4.1 per million per year, with more than 70% presenting with isolated bone disease.[52] Although LCH can occur in any bone, the most common presentation of LCH is a unifocal lesion of the skull, presenting as a painful swelling in the scalp. LCH in the head and neck can also present as painful swelling of the jaw, ear pain due to lytic destruction of the temporal bone, neck pain due to cervical vertebrae involvement and/or lymph node enlargement, and dental abnormalities. Indeed, with isolated bone disease, it is estimated that bony structures of the head and neck are involved in up to 55% of cases.[53] Although unifocal bone disease is the most common presentation, LCH can manifest as multiorgan disease of the skin (including the scalp), liver, lungs, and CNS (particularly the pituitary gland). LCH treatment is largely dependent on the site(s) of involvement at presentation. For unifocal bone disease, surgical curettage with intralesional steroid injection is usually definitive treatment, with excellent cure rates and low risk of recurrence. In multifocal bone disease or multisystem disease, systemic chemotherapy is indicated. Systemic treatment is also indicated in patients with LCH with CNS "risk lesions" (eg, extension from the skull into the CNS and/or primary CNS lesions), as they are at risk for developing diabetes insipidus and neurologic disorders both during and after treatment. Systemic chemotherapy for LCH consists of prednisone and vinblastine for 1 year. This regimen is successful in curing up to 84% of patients, with response to therapy after 12 weeks of initial treatment being an important prognostic factor.[54] Although up to 25% of patients can have a reactivation and/or refractory disease, the current recommended treatment has significantly decreased reactivation rates when compared with previous regimens.[54]

Although common in adults, SCCs of the head and neck are rare in children. Although accounting for only 1% of all pediatric tumors, SCC makes up almost 50% of all tumors of the nasopharynx in children.[55] SCC of the nasopharynx in children has been associated with EBV infection, and differing incidences by ethnicity and geography.[55,56] Presentation is usually painless lymphadenopathy, but other symptoms can include nasal obstruction, headache, otalgia, and cranial nerve involvement.[55] Standard treatment is largely based on adult experiences, but generally involves neoadjuvant cisplatin therapy and radiation therapy, followed up with adjuvant cisplatin and 5-flourouracil. Variations to this regimen have included epirubicin and bleomycin, although improved efficacy of the addition of these agents in children has not been established. OS from case series ranged from 31% to 91%, with notable improvements in survival with the addition of chemotherapy versus radiation alone.[55,56]

Late Effects

As survival rates for pediatric malignancies have improved, the long-term consequences of cancer treatments are becoming apparent in survivors. Table 1 summarizes notable late effects due to chemotherapy used in the treatment of head and neck cancers. Late effects of chemotherapy can be exacerbated by morbidity from previous surgical and radiation therapies. In addition to active surveillance for recurrence of disease, it is critical that providers coordinate efforts to monitor aggressively for late effects in their patients. Ideally, long-term monitoring would take place annually at an established cancer survivorship clinic. Guidelines for monitoring late effects of treatments for pediatric malignancies, including treatments for head and neck cancers, have been published by the COG.[19] It is critical that providers be familiar with these guidelines, as several late effects can carry severe morbidity and mortality, particularly cardiotoxicity from anthracyclines and the cumulative risk of secondary malignancies from chemotherapy and radiation exposure.[57] Finally, as the risks of late effects from treatment for pediatric malignancies can occur years to decades after treatment, proper transitioning to adult providers is critical. Discussions of transition to adult providers familiar with the care of cancer survivors should occur early, and be considered a process rather than a discrete event.[58] Evidence suggests providing detailed treatment summaries and survivor care plans will increase the likelihood of pediatric cancer survivors undergoing appropriate late effects surveillance as adults.[59,60]

SUMMARY

Cancers of the head and neck in children represent a heterogeneous group of malignancies whose successful treatment requires close coordination among a multidisciplinary team composed of a pediatric oncologist, surgeons, dentists, radiation oncologists, and a supportive care team. Although treatment with surgery, chemotherapy, and in certain cases radiation therapy has improved cure rates, these treatments have potential acute and chronic morbidities for patients of all ages. Knowledge of the acute and chronic complications of chemotherapy is critical by providers so as to support patients during treatment and throughout their lives as they transition into adult long-term survivors.

REFERENCES

1. Albright JT, Topham AK, Reilly JS. Pediatric head and neck malignancies: US incidence and trends over 2 decades. Arch Otolaryngol Head Neck Surg 2002;128(6):655–9.
2. Gosepath J, Spix C, Talebloo B, et al. Incidence of childhood cancer of the head and neck in Germany. Ann Oncol 2007;18(10):1716–21.

3. Cesmebasi A, Gabriel A, Niku D, et al. Pediatric head and neck tumors: an intra-demographic analysis using the SEER* database. Med Sci Monit 2014;20:2536–42.

4. Ries Lag SM, Gurney JG, Linet M, et al, editors. Cancer incidence and survival among children and adolescents: United States SEER program 1975–1995. Bethesda, MD: National Cancer Institute, SEER Program; 1999.

5. Ward E, DeSantis C, Robbins A, et al. Childhood and adolescent cancer statistics, 2014. CA Cancer J Clin 2014;64(2):83–103.

6. Dickson PV, Davidoff AM. Malignant neoplasms of the head and neck. Semin Pediatr Surg 2006; 15(2):92–8.

7. La Quaglia MP. Non-Hodgkin's lymphoma of the head and neck in childhood. Semin Pediatr Surg 1994;3(3):207–15.

8. Rapidis AD, Keramidas T, Panagiotopoulos H, et al. Tumours of the head and neck in the elderly: analysis of 190 patients. J Craniomaxillofac Surg 1998; 26(3):153–8.

9. Sengupta S, Pal R. Clinicopathological correlates of pediatric head and neck cancer. J Cancer Res Ther 2009;5(3):181–5.

10. Campo E, Swerdlow SH, Harris NL, et al. The 2008 WHO classification of lymphoid neoplasms and beyond: evolving concepts and practical applications. Blood 2011;117(19):5019–32.

11. Murphy SB. Classification, staging and end results of treatment of childhood non-Hodgkin's lymphomas: dissimilarities from lymphomas in adults. Semin Oncol 1980;7(3):332–9.

12. Patte C, Auperin A, Gerrard M, et al. Results of the randomized international FAB/LMB96 trial for intermediate risk B-cell non-Hodgkin lymphoma in children and adolescents: it is possible to reduce treatment for the early responding patients. Blood 2007;109(7):2773–80.

13. Burkhardt B, Zimmermann M, Oschlies I, et al. The impact of age and gender on biology, clinical features and treatment outcome of non-Hodgkin lymphoma in childhood and adolescence. Br J Haematol 2005;131(1):39–49.

14. Mbulaiteye SM, Biggar RJ, Bhatia K, et al. Sporadic childhood Burkitt lymphoma incidence in the United States during 1992–2005. Pediatr Blood Cancer 2009;53(3):366–70.

15. Reiter A, Klapper W. Recent advances in the understanding and management of diffuse large B-cell lymphoma in children. Br J Haematol 2008;142(3):329–47.

16. Sandlund JT, Downing JR, Crist WM. Non-Hodgkin's lymphoma in childhood. N Engl J Med 1996; 334(19):1238–48.

17. Yoshihara S, Nakaya M, Ichikawa T. T-cell lymphoblastic lymphoma in a child presenting as rapid

18. Reiter A, Schrappe M, Ludwig WD, et al. Intensive ALL-type therapy without local radiotherapy provides a 90% event-free survival for children with T-cell lymphoblastic lymphoma: a BFM group report. Blood 2000;95(2):416–21.

19. Children's Oncology Group. Long-term follow-up guidelines for survivors of childhood, adolescent and young adult cancers, version 4.0. Monrovia, CA: Children's Oncology Group 2013.

20. Falini B, Pileri S, Zinzani PL, et al. ALK+ lymphoma: clinico-pathological findings and outcome. Blood 1999;93(8):2697–706.

21. Stein H, Foss HD, Durkop H, et al. CD30(+) anaplastic large cell lymphoma: a review of its histopathologic, genetic, and clinical features. Blood 2000;96(12):3681–95.

22. Rosolen A, Pillon M, Garaventa A, et al. Anaplastic large cell lymphoma treated with a leukemia-like therapy: report of the Italian Association of Pediatric Hematology and Oncology (AIEOP) LNH-92 protocol. Cancer 2005;104(10):2133–40.

23. Pillon M, Gregucci F, Lombardi A, et al. Results of AIEOP LNH-97 protocol for the treatment of anaplastic large cell lymphoma of childhood. Pediatr Blood Cancer 2012;59(5):828–33.

24. Lowe EJ, Sposto R, Perkins SL, et al. Intensive chemotherapy for systemic anaplastic large cell lymphoma in children and adolescents: final results of Children's Cancer Group Study 5941. Pediatr Blood Cancer 2009;52(3):335–9.

25. Yung L, Linch D. Hodgkin's lymphoma. Lancet 2003; 361(9361):943–51.

26. Guermazi A, Brice P, de Kerviler EE, et al. Extranodal Hodgkin disease: spectrum of disease. Radiographics 2001;21(1):161–79.

27. Carbone PP, Kaplan HS, Musshoff K, et al. Report of the Committee on Hodgkin's disease staging classification. Cancer Res 1971;31(11):1860–1.

28. Metzger ML, Weinstein HJ, Hudson MM, et al. Association between radiotherapy vs no radiotherapy based on early response to VAMP chemotherapy and survival among children with favorable-risk Hodgkin lymphoma. JAMA 2012;307(24):2609–16.

29. Tebbi CK, Mendenhall NP, London WB, et al. Response-dependent and reduced treatment in lower risk Hodgkin lymphoma in children and adolescents, results of P9426: a report from the Children's Oncology Group. Pediatr Blood Cancer 2012;59(7):1259–65.

30. Wolden SL, Chen L, Kelly KM, et al. Long-term results of CCG 5942: a randomized comparison of chemotherapy with and without radiotherapy for children with Hodgkin's lymphoma–a report from the Children's Oncology Group. J Clin Oncol 2012;30(26):3174–80.

31. Dorffel W, Luders H, Ruhl U, et al. Preliminary results of the multicenter trial GPOH-HD 95 for the

treatment of Hodgkin's disease in children and adolescents: analysis and outlook. Klin Padiatr 2003; 215(3):139–45.

32. Pappo AS, Shapiro DN, Crist WM, et al. Biology and therapy of pediatric rhabdomyosarcoma. J Clin Oncol 1995;13(8):2123–39.

33. Turner JH, Richmon JD. Head and neck rhabdomyosarcoma: a critical analysis of population-based incidence and survival data. Otolaryngol Head Neck Surg 2011;145(6):967–73.

34. Breneman JC, Lyden E, Pappo AS, et al. Prognostic factors and clinical outcomes in children and adolescents with metastatic rhabdomyosarcoma–a report from the Intergroup Rhabdomyosarcoma Study IV. J Clin Oncol 2003;21(1):78–84.

35. Maurer HM, Gehan EA, Beltangady M, et al. The Intergroup Rhabdomyosarcoma Study-II. Cancer 1993;71(5):1904–22.

36. Womer RB, Daller RT, Fenton JG, et al. Granulocyte colony stimulating factor permits dose intensification by interval compression in the treatment of Ewing's sarcomas and soft tissue sarcomas in children. Eur J Cancer 2000;36(1):87–94.

37. Raney B, Anderson J, Breneman J, et al. Results in patients with cranial parameningeal sarcoma and metastases (Stage 4) treated on Intergroup Rhabdomyosarcoma Study Group (IRSG) Protocols II-IV, 1978–1997: report from the Children's Oncology Group. Pediatr Blood Cancer 2008;51(1):17–22.

38. Raney RB, Walterhouse DO, Meza JL, et al. Results of the Intergroup Rhabdomyosarcoma Study Group D9602 protocol, using vincristine and dactinomycin with or without cyclophosphamide and radiation therapy, for newly diagnosed patients with low-risk embryonal rhabdomyosarcoma: a report from the Soft Tissue Sarcoma Committee of the Children's Oncology Group. J Clin Oncol 2011;29(10):1312–8.

39. Arndt CA, Hawkins DS, Meyer WH, et al. Comparison of results of a pilot study of alternating vincristine/doxorubicin/cyclophosphamide and etoposide/ifosfamide with IRS-IV in intermediate risk rhabdomyosarcoma: a report from the Children's Oncology Group. Pediatr Blood Cancer 2008; 50(1):33–6.

40. Crist WM, Anderson JR, Meza JL, et al. Intergroup rhabdomyosarcoma study-IV: results for patients with nonmetastatic disease. J Clin Oncol 2001; 19(12):3091–102.

41. Ognjanovic S, Linabery AM, Charbonneau B, et al. Trends in childhood rhabdomyosarcoma incidence and survival in the United States, 1975–2005. Cancer 2009;115(18):4218–26.

42. Maris JM, Hogarty MD, Bagatell R, et al. Neuroblastoma. Lancet 2007;369(9579):2106–20.

43. Castellote A, Vazquez E, Vera J, et al. Cervicothoracic lesions in infants and children. Radiographics 1999;19(3):583–600.

44. Vo KT, Matthay KK, Neuhaus J, et al. Clinical, biologic, and prognostic differences on the basis of primary tumor site in neuroblastoma: a report from the international neuroblastoma risk group project. J Clin Oncol 2014;32(28):3169–76.

45. London WB, Castleberry RP, Matthay KK, et al. Evidence for an age cutoff greater than 365 days for neuroblastoma risk group stratification in the Children's Oncology Group. J Clin Oncol 2005;23(27): 6459–65.

46. Baker DL, Schmidt ML, Cohn SL, et al. Outcome after reduced chemotherapy for intermediate-risk neuroblastoma. N Engl J Med 2010;363(14): 1313–23.

47. Matthay KK, Reynolds CP, Seeger RC, et al. Long-term results for children with high-risk neuroblastoma treated on a randomized trial of myeloablative therapy followed by 13-cis-retinoic acid: a children's oncology group study. J Clin Oncol 2009;27(7): 1007–13.

48. Haddad M, Triglia JM, Helardot P, et al. Localized cervical neuroblastoma: prevention of surgical complications. Int J Pediatr Otorhinolaryngol 2003; 67(12):1361–7.

49. Qureshi SS, Kembhavi S, Ramadwar M, et al. Outcome and morbidity of surgical resection of primary cervical and cervicothoracic neuroblastoma in children: a comparative analysis. Pediatr Surg Int 2014;30(3):267–73.

50. Shields CL, Shields JA. Basic understanding of current classification and management of retinoblastoma. Curr Opin Ophthalmol 2006;17(3):228–34.

51. Finger PT, Harbour JW, Karcioglu ZA. Risk factors for metastasis in retinoblastoma. Surv Ophthalmol 2002;47(1):1–16.

52. Salotti JA, Nanduri V, Pearce MS, et al. Incidence and clinical features of Langerhans cell histiocytosis in the UK and Ireland. Arch Dis Child 2009;94(5): 376–80.

53. Hicks J, Flaitz CM. Langerhans cell histiocytosis: current insights in a molecular age with emphasis on clinical oral and maxillofacial pathology practice. Oral Surg Oral Med Oral Pathol Oral Radiol Endod 2005;100(2 Suppl I):S42–66.

54. Gadner H, Minkov M, Grois N, et al. Therapy prolongation improves outcome in multisystem Langerhans cell histiocytosis. Blood 2013;121(25): 5006–14.

55. Ayan I, Kaytan E, Ayan N. Childhood nasopharyngeal carcinoma: from biology to treatment. Lancet Oncol 2003;4(1):13–21.

56. Marcus KJ, Tishler RB. Head and neck carcinomas across the age spectrum: epidemiology, therapy, and late effects. Semin Radiat Oncol 2010;20(1): 52–7.

57. Choi DK, Helenowski I, Hijiya N. Secondary malignancies in pediatric cancer survivors: perspectives

and review of the literature. Int J Cancer 2014; 135(8):1764–73.

58. Freyer DR. Transition of care for young adult survivors of childhood and adolescent cancer: rationale and approaches. J Clin Oncol 2010;28(32):4810–8.

59. Nathan PC, Greenberg ML, Ness KK, et al. Medical care in long-term survivors of childhood cancer: a

report from the childhood cancer survivor study. J Clin Oncol 2008;26(27):4401–9.

60. Nathan PC, Ness KK, Mahoney MC, et al. Screening and surveillance for second malignant neoplasms in adult survivors of childhood cancer: a report from the childhood cancer survivor study. Ann Intern Med 2010;153(7):442–51.

Index

Note: Page numbers of article titles are in **boldface** type.

A

B

C

D

E

Oral Maxillofacial Surg Clin N Am 28 (2016) 139–144
http://dx.doi.org/10.1016/S1042-3699(15)00119-3
1042-3699/16/$ – see front matter © 2016 Elsevier Inc. All rights reserved.

Moving?

Make sure your subscription moves with you!

To notify us of your new address, find your **Clinics Account Number** (located on your mailing label above your name), and contact customer service at:

Email: journalscustomerservice-usa@elsevier.com

800-654-2452 (subscribers in the U.S. & Canada)
314-447-8871 (subscribers outside of the U.S. & Canada)

Fax number: 314-447-8029

**Elsevier Health Sciences Division
Subscription Customer Service
3251 Riverport Lane
Maryland Heights, MO 63043**

*To ensure uninterrupted delivery of your subscription, please notify us at least 4 weeks in advance of move.